MW00637875

The New Alkaline Diet Cookbook 2021

Beginners Edition

© Copyright 2021
All rights reserved.

This document is geared towards providing exact and reliable information with regards to the topic and issue covered. The publication is sold with the idea that the publisher is not required to render accounting, officially permitted, or otherwise, qualified services. If advice is necessary, legal or professional, a practiced individual in the profession should be ordered.

- From a Declaration of Principles which was accepted and approved equally by a Committee of the American Bar Association and a Committee of Publishers and Associations.

In no way is it legal to reproduce, duplicate, or transmit any part of this document in either electronic means or in printed format. Recording of this publication is strictly prohibited and any storage of this document is not allowed unless with written permission from the publisher. All rights reserved.

The information provided herein is stated to be truthful and consistent, in that any liability, in terms of inattention or otherwise, by any usage or abuse of any policies, processes, or directions contained within is the solitary and utter responsibility of the recipient reader. Under no circumstances will any legal responsibility or blame be held against the publisher for any reparation, damages, or monetary loss due to the information herein, either directly or indirectly.

Respective authors own all copyrights not held by
the publisher.

The information herein is offered for informational
purposes solely, and is universal as so. The
presentation of the information is without contract
or any type of guarantee assurance.
The trademarks that are used are without any consent, and
the publication of the trademark is without permission or
backing by the trademark owner. All trademarks and
brands within this book are for clarifying purposes only and
are the owned by the owners themselves, not affiliated with
this document.

Table of Contents

Avocado Pesto Zoodles

filled pumpkin

Stir-fry   vegetables

Avocado - potato salad

Ideal for in between - 4 basic snack recipes

Basic chocolate mousse

Vegetable chips

Beetroot cream

Cashew spread

Always ready - 43 other basic recipes ideal for basic cures

Special kale salad

Curry pan with potatoes

Almond milk shake

Potato dumplings

kohlrabi soup

The special dressing

Mediterranean vegetables from the oven

Eggplant rolls with basil

KiBa - smoothie

Basic dressing

Soup made from nettles

Chili pumpkin

Turmeric smoothie

Millet porridge

Millet   porridge

Basic breakfast cereal

Purslane salad

Thai quinoa salad

Buckwheat   porridge

Fennel soup with zucchini

Broccoli Salad with Quinoa

Vegetables from the oven

Quinoa and carrot salad

Carrot Millet Bread

Basic stuffed peppers

Vegan couscous salad

Corn salad smoothie

Preface

Alkaline nutrition this is a topic that more and more people are dealing with. This type of diet promises a better and much healthier lifestyle. But what is it actually about in detail?
In short - in an alkaline diet, a person consumes basic minerals and the essential nutrients to keep the body in optimal balance. This avoids acidic metabolic residues. The goal is simply that the acid-base balance is balanced. Life will be a lot easier as a result.

The following chapters explain in detail what alkaline nutrition actually is and why it is so good for general well-being. It is also explained about acidosis and which foods should and should not go into the shopping basket.
Thus, there are also many delicious recipes for an alkaline diet, developed for every taste. Not only are they easy and inexpensive to prepare, they but also offer a lot of variety in everyday life. And it will definitely fill you up - that's guaranteed.
Become an expert in alkaline nutrition - in just 10 days!

The emergence of the alkaline diet

The first theses on this topic were put forward as early as the middle of the 17th century. It was believed that an unbalanced acid-base balance in the body can lead to serious illnesses. This was initially claimed by Francis de la Boe Sylvius, but he related his statements to the humors. Acids and alkalis were then prescribed to treat this imbalance.
It was not until the beginning of the 20th century that this theory was revisited by Howard Hay and Franz Xaver Mayr. The quote "The acid is the ultimate cell poison." arose from it.

The theory only became famous later through a Swedish scientist who did all kinds of research on the subject. He discovered the so-called "excess acid" and suspected that it could even lead to death. The reason for this, however, was that he brought acidification directly into connection with diabetes. As we know today, this assumption was wrong.
A little later, Bircher-Benner formulated the following thesis: "If the excess acid increases so high that the food bases are no longer sufficient, the organism gradually becomes acidic." The consequences of this then extended to life-threatening acid poisoning.
In 1927, a book about hyperacidity was published for the first time, written by the American doctor Alfred McCann namely "Cultural Disease and Acid Death". It dealt with the exact same theory. Excessive consumption of meat was considered to be the reason for too much acid in the body, which then had to be excreted through the kidneys. Meat eaters were therefore provocatively referred to as kidney killers in the book. A somewhat exaggerated statement. McCann almost despised meat eaters even if it was actually his friends.

The researcher, Berg also made clear progress in his studies on alkaline nutrition. He knew that tubers and vegetables are almost the only carriers of bases, but that they would lose them again through cooking and draining. He advised the consumption of raw vegetables - for example in the form of a delicious salad. The beginnings of the alkaline diet were now born.

All previous scientists assumed that ammonia was a very harmful metabolic waste product, but this theory soon turned out to be completely wrong. Ammonia was much more an end product of our body's metabolism and helpful in eliminating acidic protons. A special form of protein is created from supposedly acidic and also basic foods.

At that time, Ragnar Berg saw in the acid generator only waste products - also known as waste products - of the body. They were considered harmful and had to leave the body quickly. These waste products result from a high-acid or low-base diet and can lead to various metabolic diseases. You have to eat more and still get less energy. With a diet rich in bases, however, the energy is passed on from the food to the body in the best possible way. Less slag is formed.

The disadvantage of Berg's theory, however, was that more and more substances in the body were subsequently declared to be waste products and had to be removed again using supposed miracle cures. Pure greed for profit and less for the benefit of health.

What is an alkaline diet?

The origins of the alkaline diet have now been clearly clarified. But there is still a whole new question to answer:
What exactly is the alkaline diet?
However, this is very easy to explain, because this form of nutrition simply refers to the consumption of alkaline foods. Food that forms acid, on the other hand, is strictly avoided.
An alkaline diet prevents over-acidification - this is harmful and can lead to some diseases of the body. If there is already over-acidification, this can also be reduced by the alkaline diet.
A balanced acid-base balance can be named as a general goal. Incidentally, only corpses are naturally acidic - and of course you don't necessarily want to be one of them.
An alkaline diet is said to bring you a longer life. The secret is the perfect pH value anytime and anywhere.
PH value? What's this?

Many people may have heard of it before, because this value indicates how much alkaline or acid something is. The pH value scale ranges from 1-14. The first seven values are acidic and all others are basic. The 7 itself is the neutral number.
But watch out - if the body is over-acidic, this does not mean that it only has to have values below 7. Thinking is the mistake of most people. In the case of over-acidification, there is a disruption of the acid-base balance. Exactly this means that normally basic parts of the body have too much acid. The opposite can also be the case - naturally acidic parts of the body suddenly have an increased pH value.
As an example of this, one can take the body's blood. It should always be basic. Incidentally, this also applies to the fluids in the bile and the connective tissue. However, there should always be a slightly acidic atmosphere in the large intestine in a healthy person. The same applies to the stomach and genital organs of women.

The aim of an alkaline diet is therefore not to increase the pH of the entire body. That would be at least as damaging as hyperacidity. The goal is simply to deacidify evenly and in a controlled manner. A deacidification program is often included for this purpose. In this way, all areas of the body that require a basic pH value are optimally supplied.

Incidentally, the alkaline diet also helps regulate gastric acid production. A balance is established. It also allows beneficial bacteria to create a better natural - and acidic - environment in the colon and vagina.

The acid-base balance in detail

With an alkaline diet, everything really depends on the acid-base balance of the body. It has to be in balance so that well-being and health are optimal. It has already been explained a bit how this acid-base balance works, but now the details come - because nothing is more important than to understand the whole method correctly before you eat an alkaline diet.

The acid-base balance is sometimes just called the base balance and consists of several different buffer systems. They ensure that fluctuations in the pH values in the body are balanced out. Additional bases are absorbed and acids are excreted - according to the needs of the health. Of course, the whole thing can work in exactly the opposite way.
According to the buffer systems, it is very important to distinguish between them. There are open and closed buffer systems. The open systems transport the acids and bases out of the body when they are in the majority. The best known is the bicarbonate buffer system. It breathes the substances out of the lungs in the form of carbon dioxide. Then there is the ammonium buffer system - it excretes acids through the urinary tract.
The closed buffer systems, on the other hand, work differently, because both bases and acids remain in the body. However, they are bound and can be better controlled and regulated. The protein buffer system is a good example. Among other things, it absorbs hemoglobin - a red blood pigment. The substances are then bound to this.

How exactly it looks in the acid-base balance is best determined by a doctor. He can also check the blood gas values at the same time. There is also a control over the functions of the heart, lungs, the buffer systems and especially the kidneys. Disturbances in this organ particularly affect the acid-base balance.
During the entire examination, it is very important that the doctor understands this topic very well, because the results must be interpreted correctly. There are metabolic or lung disorders - metabolic or respiratory disorders. First, the body tries to compensate for these irregularities by itself.

In order to precisely check all values, a doctor often only needs a small sample of the blood. It certainly doesn't hurt either. A special method is then used to assess the balance, but it can also be very complicated. The pH value is also compared with the average values at the end. In normal adults, it is between 7.36 and 7.44. By the way, children have different norms.

If the pH values in the body are too low, this is called acidosis so it is considered the acidity. Moreover, the worst case that can occur is when both the levels of carbon dioxide are increased and those of the biocarbonate are too low. Multiple organ failure can occur.

If too many bases are found in the blood, one speaks of an alkalosis. This is exactly the opposite of acidosis. The causes for this are usually stress, disorders of the kidney functions or frequent vomiting.

No matter how the acid-base balance is disturbed, it often regulates itself again. That's what the buffer systems are for. But even beyond that, there are several steps that can help restore balance.
If the disorders and the symptoms are particularly severe, the reason for them should be found quickly. If hyperventilation occurs - due to a disturbed acid-base balance - certain breathing techniques should be used. Insulin helps with diabetes.

The decisive advantages of an alkaline diet

Of course, the base-rich diet has many other advantages to offer, which affect the body and to a certain extent the mind. Especially if you are not quite sure whether you want to try this form of nutrition, it is always worth taking a look at the pluses that the alkaline diet brings for the whole body.
An alkaline diet is more than a way of eating - it is a diverse lifestyle.
You can make light fat deposits disappear, improve the complexion and get more energy in everyday life. Generally you feel much better.
But let's start from the beginning and all the advantages explained in detail:

Fat disappears

Sounds almost like a diet, but it is meant a little differently. When the body is acidic, acids and toxins are bound to fat. Accumulations of water can also occur. So if you have too much fat on your hips, this can also be a sign of too much acid in the body.
If the acid-base balance of the body is brought back into balance by minerals, the body no longer necessarily needs the fat and water. An alkaline diet breaks down slags very easily and weight is automatically reduced at the same time. Problem areas can disappear.

More beautiful skin

Reducing weight is one thing. At the same time, an alkaline diet can also significantly improve the complexion. Conventional diets do not have this advantage, but this form of nutrition firms and cleanses the connective tissue of the skin in the long term. In addition, this effect can also be intensified with an alkaline skin care product. The formation of autologous fat is stimulated and daily creaming will soon be superfluous.

No more cravings

Cravings can not only get on your nerves, but also go deep into your wallet. With an alkaline diet one does not forego food, but looks for healthier alternatives to the usual dishes. In this way, the body is well supplied with a rich base and a great variety. The feeling of cravings is therefore absent.

Deficiency symptoms are compensated

Diets are often designed to simply leave out certain substances. Of course, in most cases this leads to deficiency symptoms. This is different with an alkaline diet - all of the body's depots are automatically refilled. The body functions will continue to run optimally and the nasty deficiency symptoms will not occur at all. This also makes people appear healthier from the outside.

Increase energy and performance

If you use many additional products that supposedly promise a healthier life, the body is very often supplied with too few minerals. On the contrary - sometimes important nutrients are withdrawn from it.
An alkaline diet, on the other hand, brings more energy because the body is adequately supplied with minerals and vitamins. So you can get through the stressful day and see a lot more relaxed.

Perception of fellow human beings improves

Of course, the main focus of an alkaline diet is on the physical changes, but much more is happening in the background. The environment simply perceives you differently - or more positively. One feels internally balanced and is more resilient for the stony paths of life. The body looks taut and the complexion shinier - other people see that too. The effect is clearly more positive.

Mental sharpness

Artificial products are now a thing of the past, so after a while you will feel a lot livelier spiritually. The "brain smog" - the familiar foggy feeling in the head disappears completely and the thoughts become faster again.

Whoever does everything the same in life and doesn't dare to do anything new can never change anything. Regardless of whether you are in a mental or physical state - everything will stay the same. Sometimes it's just a small change that brings real miracles.
The alkaline diet is definitely a big step in the right direction. It is not only healthy, but also offers many delicious dishes - and you can easily cook them yourself.
With an alkaline diet, you not only improve your health and balance, but also your external appearance. You don't even have to radically change your life. Switching to healthy foods step by step is enough.
In summary, you should always keep these advantages in mind:

- ☐ Fat **pads disappear**
- ☐ The complexion **becomes better**
- ☐ **Energy and performance increase**
- ☐ **No more cravings**
- ☐ There are no **deficiency symptoms**
- ☐ **Spiritual sharpness arises**
- ☐ People's **perception is positive**

In addition to all these impressive advantages, every person will surely discover more for themselves.

How does hyperacidity arise?

Acidification - what is it actually?
Over-acidification is the disruption of the acid-base balance in our
body. Usually this also leads to a drop in the pH value in the blood.
The balance between acids and bases in the body is regulated by a
complicated mechanism. It is only through it that all important metabolic
processes function.

Acidification - or other disturbances in this household - is usually caused by
various foods. Those have a higher proportion of acid.

These include, for example:

- meat
- eggs
- Pasta

Foods that counteract this are those that have a high base content. That
would be for example:

- fruit
- vegetables
- herbs

The body always tries to keep the acid-base balance in perfect balance,
because it reacts extremely sensitively to fluctuations.
The body naturally achieves this balance through gas exchange in the lungs,
through the buffering properties of tissue and blood, and the excretory
mechanisms of the kidney. But if these do not work properly or are
exhausted, too many acidic components enter the blood and over-
acidification can occur.

Experts refer to this acidosis as acidosis - a disorder in which the pH value
in the body falls below 7.35.

The reason for this is often an incorrect or poorly considered diet. But if you are completely healthy, then food has little influence on the acid-base balance, because the buffer systems do their job excellently and the pH value remains constant.

Incidentally, the pH value has an important meaning for our whole body. It decides on many metabolic processes.

These are among others:

- ☐ the work of the heart muscle
- ☐ the sugar metabolism
- ☐ the formation of oxygen

The abbreviation pH stands for "potentia Hydrogenii". This comes from the Latin and stands for "concentration of hydrogen. The value actually indicates how many ions of hydrogen are in a liquid. The blood of a healthy person has a pH value of 7.4. The value is based on a special blood gas analysis and gives precise information about a potential health disorder.

As already mentioned, the buffer systems in the body are used for regulation primarily in the blood and urine. The protein in particular has a great effect, because it has the property of binding excess hydrogen ions and sometimes even excreting them.

If these buffer systems are no longer sufficient - you eat unhealthily for a very long time and with too little base-forming foods - then at some point chronic acidosis can also occur. Of course, this also has fatal consequences, which unfortunately often go unnoticed.

This could be an example:

- ☐ Tissues and organs are attacked and this leads to further diseases and chronic complaints.
- ☐ Acid provides the perfect atmosphere for harmful bacteria. They can then affect entire organs.

□ Almost every vital function can be significantly impaired. Acidification is the cause of many diseases and complaints that can also become chronic.

□ The symptoms of hyperacidity are often quite different and unspecific. No uniform picture is perceived because normal pain, tiredness or, for example, heartburn can occur.

□ Dandruff, hair loss, bad breath or unclean skin can be other signs of acidosis.

□ Acidification is the perfect starting point for many other diseases. These include osteoporosis, migraines, diabetes and gout.

□ Another notable consequence of hyperacidity is obesity. Incidentally, this can also be viewed as a symptom of the disorder.

So that it doesn't get that far in the first place, you should prevent over-acidification of the body beforehand. Much more than a lot of discipline is not necessary - and a few tips that will reduce the risk of hyperacidity within a few weeks. This is how you ultimately avoid the unpleasant consequences and diseases.

Here are 5 simple tips that really everyone can integrate perfectly into their everyday life:

1. Change of diet
Acidic foods - such as meat or sweets must be avoided. An alkaline diet is now on the agenda. This includes fruits, vegetables as well as drinking plenty of pure water.

2. Basic minerals
However, do not overdo it, because when the acid-base balance is back in equilibrium that can also be harmful. Alkaline minerals replenish the natural buffer systems in the blood and help even after an intensive cure with an alkaline diet.

3. Base baths
These are baths that you can indulge in for an hour 2-3 times a week. Special alkaline bath additives are used for this. You can

enjoy this bath as a foot bath or a full bath - entirely as you wish. Here, too, the blood buffers are balanced again and harmful waste products are excreted. As an addition, you can also be massaged with a brush, because this reactivates the lymphatic system.

4. Much sport
Even a little regular exercise can bring the acid-base balance back into balance. Proper sweating helps a lot more, of course. Too much exertion, on the other hand, is harmful again, because it can lead to unhealthy overload.

5. Relaxation is a must
Unfortunately, in everyday life you are often stressed yourself, but it is precisely then that you should treat yourself to small moments of rest from time to time. This includes relaxed eating and adequate sleep. Negative thoughts should be avoided. Yoga or meditation can be very helpful here.

The right foods in an alkaline diet

Basic foods are definitely part of an alkaline diet.

But what is it actually?

This includes all foods that the body converts into bases. The explanation for this can be found in biochemistry. There, the individual foods are assessed according to how many proteins, fats or carbohydrates they contain - and whether they have an alkaline or acidic effect.

Many studies in recent years have shown that alkaline foods have a better long-term effect on human health. The researcher, Ragnar Berg recommended in his theory at the time to consume around five times more foods that form bases than those that are converted into acid.

In order for a food to become basic, it must have a high proportion of basic minerals. These include potassium, magnesium and calcium. However, protein should not be found in excessive amounts. This largely includes fruit, vegetables and herbs.

Potassium plays the biggest role here - often in the form of potassium salts or potassium citrate - but the other minerals also have a major influence. The proportion of these substances in a food then gives the final base proportion. There are special acid-base tables for this purpose. These are just kept simple, because there are many more substances that have an influence on the acid-base value of food. The 100% determination of the acid content is very complicated and has not yet been included in any calculation.

However, one should not only pay attention to the high potassium content in food because that would be a big mistake. One-sided nutrition is not exactly healthy either.

Foods in an alkaline diet have several points in common, first and foremost that they have an alkaline effect. But they also contain hardly any protein and are mostly vegetable - fruits and vegetables. There are only a few exceptions.

In general, these foods are best suited:

- **vegetables**
- **fruit**
- **herbs**
- **mushrooms**
- **seedlings**
- **seeds**
- **Cores**
- **Almonds**
- **walnuts**
- **pistachios**
- **Macadamia nuts**

Foods are taboo

Acidification is harmful. Not only does it make you seriously ill, it but also makes you fat. That is already a fact. In addition, the organs are stressed and fungi and harmful bacteria settle better. The alkaline diet fights against this, is delicious and offers a lot of variety.
There is also something in the alkaline diet for lovers of sweets and small snacks, because there are also special cakes and even ice cream.

But it is also the case that you should absolutely avoid some foods because they form too much acid. Acidification can be the result.
These products should therefore be avoided in an alkaline diet:

- **alcohol**
- **Soft drinks**
- **sausage**
- **eggs**
- **jam**
- **Quark**
- **nicotine**

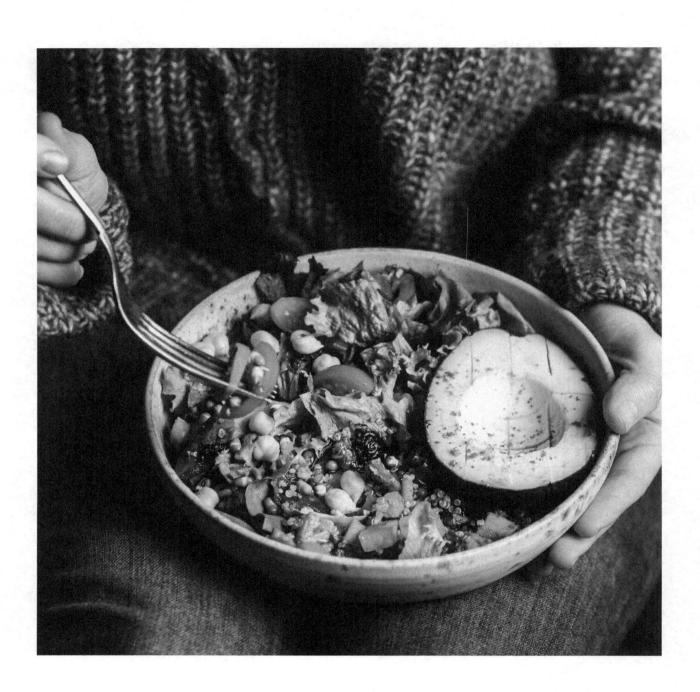

65 optimal and delicious recipes

The alkaline diet is not only a real treat for the body - but also for the mind and soul. The best thing about it is that it never gets boring or tasteless, because there are a multitude of recipes and there is definitely something for everyone.
In general, one can say that the alkaline diet is very similar to the vegan diet, as animal products are largely avoided. That is also clear, because they form acid. In contrast, fruits, vegetables and many fresh herbs are used. But what is the difference to vegan cuisine?
Quite simply - the alkaline diet aims to bring the acid-base balance of the body back into the right balance.

The main components of the delicious dishes are the alkaline foods. 80% of them belong in the food. As a supplement, you can then add small acid-forming products - for example whole grains or nuts.
Vegetable soups are simple and suitable for this. They don't do that much work and you can use just about any variety. Simply peel and cut the vegetables if necessary and then cook them in a broth (based on alkaline). Puree at the end and you have a wholesome soup.
However, you shouldn't make the mistake of adding dairy products to taste. They are namely poison in the alkaline diet. How about some healthy vegetable oils? These oils still give a dish that certain something.
Many herbs are also very important for seasoning - fresh ones. Here you can be creative at your own discretion. Trying something new has never hurt anyone.
A tip - almond or nut pastes have a similar taste to cream and can perfectly season a dish.
With all this, however, you should also make sure that no sugar is used, otherwise the alkaline effect will quickly be over. Fortunately, there are many suitable alternatives for this that is less unhealthy.

A real alkaline diet starts with breakfast. Unfortunately, many people eat unhealthy foods early in the day - cornflakes and sweet rolls are just two small examples. Even cheese is taboo in this form of diet.

This should also be avoided:
- coffee
- Products made from milk
- Nutella
- eggs
- Bakery products

Water can always be drunk. But since many people don't find it very tasty, it can also be refined. Herbs or even a small wedge of lemon can really help. But sugar shouldn't be used here either.

Now back to the basic breakfast. This consists largely of fruit and vegetables, but can also contain small amounts of nuts or whole grains.

That would be for example:
- juices
- smoothies
- raw food

That was enough of the preface. Here are the best and most delicious recipes for a healthy and alkaline breakfast!

7 delicious breakfast ideas
Chard and thyme smoothie

A smoothie is always a good alternative to solid food. The green varieties in particular are not only extremely healthy, they also taste really good. Many nutrients - such as vitamins and calcium - are included here.

ingredients

- 100 grams of Swiss chard
- 1 apple
- 1 pear
- 2 stalks of thyme
- 1 banana
- 500 ml of lime juice

preparation

Firstly, wash and chop the chard, then wash off the fruit (apple and pear), remove the stones and cut into cubes. Now wash the thyme and pluck carefully the leaves from the stems.
Put everything together with the banana, the lime juice and 300 ml of water in the blender and puree well. You can use more water if you like.

Avocado smoothie

Avocados - these are the perfect basic foods. This smoothie is also rich in minerals and healthy fats.

ingredients

- 1 avocado
- 1 banana
- 1 handful of spinach
- 300 ml of water

preparation

First, the avocado has to be halved, the pits removed and the skin removed. Then you have to peel the banana. Now cut everything into small pieces and put in the blender. Cut the washed spinach into small pieces and add to the water. Mix everything again.

The super green smoothie

This smoothie is green again, making it a real pick-me-up for boring days. It is not only perfect for an alkaline breakfast, but is also a good snack between meals.

ingredients

- 1 avocado
- 1 half cucumber
- 1 handful of rocket
- 10 basil leaves
- 1 handful of mint leaves
- 1 papaya

preparation

At the beginning, the avocado is halved, the stone removed and peeled. Then you have to cut them into large pieces. The cucumber is now also washed and grated. The inside is cut into large pieces.
Now the leaves of the rocket, basil and mint must be washed off and sorted. Now cut open the papaya and simply core it with a spoon. Remove the flesh of the fruit and cut into pieces. Put everything in the mixer together with the water and puree.

Coconut smoothie bowl

Vegan and alkaline recipes are particularly known for the fact that they are varied and at the same time very intense in taste. They are rich in healthy energy.

ingredients

- 1 banana
- 2 kiwis
- 200 grams of pineapple
- 60 grams of spinach
- Lime juice
- 100 ml coconut milk
- 2 teaspoons of chia seeds
- 3 teaspoons of coconut flakes

preparation

First, the banana, pineapple and kiwi fruit must be peeled. With the pineapple, care must be taken to remove the woody-tasting eye. Then roughly cut everything. For decoration you should put some banana and kiwi aside.
Put the fruit - and the spinach - in the blender along with the lime juice and coconut milk and puree.
Use the remains of the banana and kiwi fruit for decoration at the end. Then add the chia seeds and the coconut flakes.

Alkaline fruit salad

Fruit salad is a standard in alkaline nutrition and also always offers an extra kick of freshness.

ingredients

- 2 nectarines
- 200 grams of strawberries
- 100 grams of gooseberries
- 4 tbsp orange juice
- 1 tbsp orange jam
- Melissa leaves

preparation

First, the nectarines are washed, dried and the stone removed. Then they are cut into thin slices. The strawberries are also washed and cleaned and then cut in half. Wash the gooseberries too.
Now the jam must be mixed with the orange juice. The fruits are put in a small bowl and the mix of juice and jam is spread over it. Then everything is carefully mixed with a spoon. Now it has to drag for about ten minutes. If necessary, you can garnish the salad with the lemon balm leaves.

Raw fruit and vegetables salad

With this salad, only very fresh vegetables come on the plate. A pleasure likes in spring.

ingredients

- 1 apple
- 2 tbsp honey
- pepper
- salt
- parsley
- 1 bunch of radishes
- 1 kohlrabi
- 1 spring onion
- 2 tbsp sunflower oil
- lemon juice

preparation

First of all, the kohlrabi, apple, spring onions and radishes need to be washed and then the apple needs to be dried. The kohlrabi is now peeled and cut into thin slices. The same is done with the radishes and the spring onions are cut into rings.
Now the parsley is chopped. Lemon juice, pepper, salt, oil and honey are mixed together to make a dressing for the salad.
Now arrange the prepared vegetables in a bowl and mix well with the dressing. At the end a little parsley is sprinkled over it for decoration.

Fruity avocado dip

A dip can also add just the right flavor to a meal, especially if it is as healthy and fruity as this avocado dip.

ingredients

- 1 avocado
- Juice from half a lime
- 2.5 drops of Tabasco
- sea salt
- 1 half mango

preparation

Loosen the pulp of the avocado and place in a small bowl. Then add the Tabasco, lime juice and sea salt. Chop the whole thing with a fork. Remove the pulp of the mango from the stone and then cut into small cubes. Add to the dip.

Breakfast is the most important meal, but lunch also plays a major role in health. In the middle of the day, you are supplied with exactly the amount of energy you need.

An alkaline lunch consists of a lot of vegetables - for example in the form of salads or soups. Herbs, nuts and tofu can also be included. As with breakfast, you should avoid dairy products. However, all dishes can be perfectly refined with healthy vegetable oils.

11 recipes for the perfect alkaline lunch

Coconut turnip soup

Something is completely different than the usual pumpkin soup. With its exotic taste and spicy curry, this turnip soup is a treat for the palate.

Ingredients:

- 600 grams of turnips
- 2 potatoes
- 2 shallots
- 1 clove of garlic
- 1 ginger
- 2 tbsp coconut oil
- 600 ml of vegetable stock
- 300 ml coconut milk
- orange juice
- anise
- Allspice
- sea salt
- 1.5 spring onions
- 3 stalks of chervil

preparation

First, peel the potatoes and turnips and cut them into cubes. Do the same with the garlic and ginger. Now heat the coconut oil in a saucepan and sweat the garlic, ginger and shallots in it.
Add the potatoes and turnips and deglaze everything with a little broth. Then there is coconut milk and the orange juice. The whole thing has to cook for about a quarter of an hour.
Finally, the soup is pureed and seasoned with curry, anise, sea salt and allspice. Only now are the spring onions cut into small rings. The soup is filled into smaller bowls and sprinkled with the spring onions and chervil for decoration.

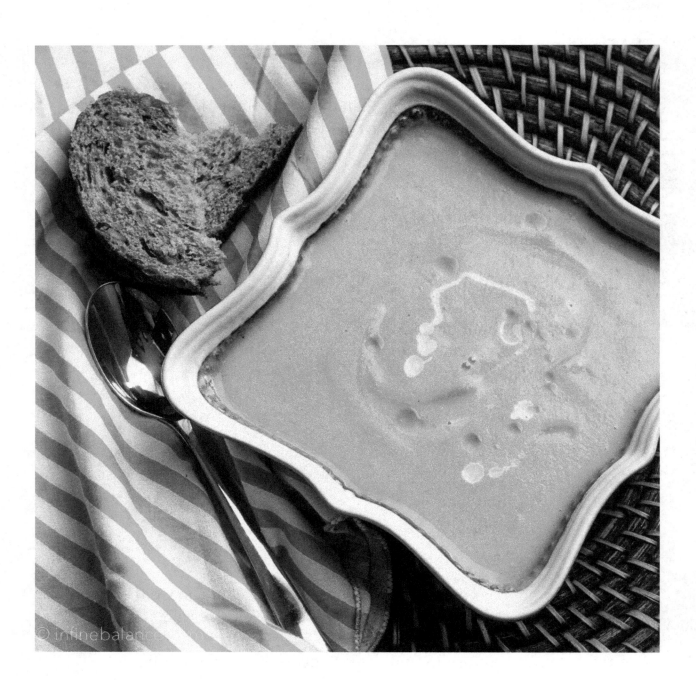

© infinebalance.com

Tomato soup

This soup is not only very low in calories, it is also particularly quick to prepare.

ingredients

- 1 can of tomatoes
- 500 ml of broth
- 2 tomatoes
- broccoli
- 100 grams of champions
- 1 half bunch of chives
- salt
- pepper

preparation

The canned tomatoes have to be drained and the tomato juice can be used for other purposes. Then they need to be cut into small pieces and heated in the broth.
The fresh tomatoes are now quartered and the broccoli divided into florets. The champions are also cleaned and then divided by four.
Put everything in the tomato stock and cook for a quarter of an hour. Now the chives - cut into rolls - are added. Finally, add salt and pepper to the dish.

Raw vegetable salad with tofu

All possible colors are represented here. This salad is not only a delight for the palate, but also beautiful to look at.

ingredients

- 300 grams of pointed cabbage
- 3 carrots
- 1 bunch of radishes
- 1 can of corn
- 1 tbsp rapeseed oil
- 400 grams of nut tofu
- 150 grams of yogurt
- 2 tablespoons of lemon juice
- 1 teaspoon olive oil
- 1 teaspoon sweet mustard
- pepper
- sea salt
- cress

preparation

The vegetables need cleaning and the carrots and cabbage grated. Celery and radishes, on the other hand, need to be cut into tender slices. Then everything is mixed with corn. Meanwhile, the oil is warmed up in the pan. Now dice the tofu and fry in it.
Now the yoghurt is mixed with the cress, the spices, the lemon juice, oil and the sweet mustard and seasoned. The salad is finally served with dressing and tofu.

Orange salad with savoy cabbage and nuts

Savoy cabbage is a vegetable that is full to the brim with important nutrients - and has next to no calories. This a must in an alkaline diet.

ingredients

- 250 grams of savoy cabbage
- 2 oranges
- 1 teaspoon olive oil
- 1 tbsp fruit vinegar
- 1 teaspoon agave syrup
- sea salt
- pepper
- 1 shallot
- basil
- 2 chopped walnuts

preparation

The savoy cabbage is cleaned and separated from the stalk. The individual leaves are then placed in boiling salted water and left there for half a minute. After that, the savoy cabbage must drain in a sieve and dry. Then it is cut into thumb-thick strips.
Then the orange is peeled and the white skin is completely removed. The fillet of orange is cut out.
Half an orange is squeezed out and the resulting juice is then mixed with the olive oil, the spices, the agave syrup and the vinegar. Now the shallot has to be peeled and diced. Then she comes to dressing. The savoy cabbage and the fillets of orange are served on a plate - drizzled with dressing. You can use basil leaves and chopped walnuts as decoration.
By the way, this salad also works well with persimmons.

Parsley salad

This dish is fruity and spicy - and full of valuable beta-carotene.

ingredients

- 2 bunches of parsley
- 3 stalks of mint
- 1 half yellow pepper
- 1 spring onion
- 1 pomegranate
- 100 grams of watermelon
- 1 half a lemon
- 3 tablespoons of olive oil
- sea salt
- black pepper

preparation

First, the herbs need to be washed and cut into strips. Then the peppers are cleaned and cut into cubes. Wash the spring onions and cut into small rings. Now the pomegranate has to be halved and squeezed. This works best with a lemon press. The other half of the pomegranate is only pitted. The melon is diced.

Now mix the lemon juice together with the zest, salt, pepper, oil and the juice of the pomegranate. Put the herbs and spring onion in a bowl with most of the dressing. Then add the peppers and fruits. Finally, drip the rest of the dressing on top.

Quinoa and avocado salad

This salad is not only particularly quick to prepare, it is also really versatile. You can use it for lunch or just for the next party. Anyone as they please.

ingredients

- 1 half avocado
- 1 tomato
- 1 half cucumber
- 1 handful of spinach
- 1 tbsp olive oil
- 1 tbsp lemon juice
- 1 teaspoon agave syrup
- salt
- pepper

preparation

First, prepare the quinoa as it says on the package insert. Then place on a plate and let cool down a little.
Now the avocado has to be cut into strips and the tomato and cucumber into cubes. Then everything is mixed with the quinoa in a bowl.
Then agave syrup, the oil, the lemon juice, salt and pepper are mixed together and added to the finished salad when serving.

Finally, at the end of the day, dinner is due. This is at least as important as the other two meals. Of course, you can also use the recipes for salads and soups for this, but often the hunger is greatest at the end of the day. Hearty dishes - which are still basic - are the better choice.

Chickpea stew from Morocco

A real vacation in Morocco is mostly all-inclusive. This is what it looks like with this particular stew. Minerals and vitamins are also included.

ingredients

- 2 cloves of garlic
- 1 onion
- 1 piece of ginger
- 1 sweet potato
- 1 bulb of fennel
- 1 half zucchini
- 1 half yellow pepper
- 1 tbsp rapeseed oil
- different spices (as you like)
- 1 half teaspoon of Chili flakes
- 1 half teaspoon of cinnamon
- sea salt
- 2 tablespoons of tomato paste
- 500 ml of vegetable stock
- 1 can of chickpeas
- 1 half bunch of parsley
- 1 half orange

preparation

Firstly, peel and chop the garlic, onion and ginger. Also, remove the skin from the sweet potato and cut into cubes. Clean and cut the peppers. The zucchini must be halved and cut into small slices.
Heat some oil in a wok and heat onion, garlic and ginger in it for about three minutes. Now add the remaining vegetables and spices and steam for another five minutes. Now add the tomato paste and the broth. The whole thing has to cook on a low heat for a quarter of an hour. At the same time wash and drain the chickpeas. Finally, mix with the vegetables and leave on the stove for another five minutes with the lid closed.

Now the parsley needs to be washed, dried and finely chopped. The whole stew is now seasoned with the orange juice and the orange peel and finally served.

Avocado Pesto Zoodles

What are zoodles again? Very simple - the latest trend in vegan and alkaline kitchens around the world. They are zucchini strips cut in the shape of spaghetti. This variant also includes the totally versatile avocado.

ingredients

- *2* zucchini
- 1 avocado
- 125 grams of frozen spinach
- 3 tbsp pine nuts
- 1 clove of garlic
- 1 half a lemon
- 6 cherry tomatoes
- 1 tbsp olive oil
- 2 tbsp rapeseed oil
- salt
- Cayenne pepper

preparation

The zucchini must first be washed. Then their ends are cut off and they are made into noodles. This works either with a spiral cutter or a vegetable peeler - depending on whether you want spaghetti or ribbon noodles.
A bowl has to be lined with paper towels and the zoodles go in there. They are sprinkled with a pinch of salt and massaged briefly. Now they need to be watered for half an hour. Then you have to squeeze out the kitchen roll and fry the zoodles for three minutes on a medium flame with a little oil. The spinach can also be thawed in the microwave, but it should not be boiled.
Now the avocado has to be halved and the stone removed. The pulp is then put in a blender. Peel and add the garlic, along with the pine nuts, juice, lemon and spinach. The whole thing is then pureed into a pesto with a creamy consistency and placed in a bowl.

Season everything with a little salt and cayenne pepper - if necessary lemon
- and serve with the warm zoodles.
You can decorate the dish with halved cherry tomatoes and other pine nuts.

filled pumpkin

This dish is not only basic, but also low-carb. So it's healthy and also helps you lose a few pounds.

ingredients

- 1 Hokkaido pumpkin
- 2 tablespoons of olive oil
- 1 onion
- 300 grams of tofu
- 300 grams of frozen spinach
- 7 tbsp plant cream
- 2 teaspoons of mustard
- Nutmeg
- black pepper
- salt
- 2 carrots
- 1 spring onion
- 2 teaspoons of sesame seeds
- 1 bunch of oregano

preparation

The pumpkin must be cut in half, and the seeds are removed with a spoon. After that, the flesh of the pumpkin is coated with oil. The halves are then placed on a baking sheet with the smooth side up. Bake in the preheated oven on the middle rack at 200-220 degrees for about half an hour.
In the meantime, cut the onion into cubes and heat in a pan with oil. Chop the tofu into pieces as wide as a thumb and add to the onions. Fry over high heat for around seven minutes - until it turns golden brown.
For the filling, heat the spinach as described on the package insert and add the tofu mixture, plant cream and mustard. Season everything with the spices.

Now the filling is spread over the finished pumpkin halves and baked again for ten minutes at 160-180 degrees.

Now comes the topping. To do this, cut the carrots into slices and the spring onions into small rings. Heat with oil in a pan. Roast the black sesame seeds briefly. Now the oregano is chopped into small pieces. This is then sprinkled over the pumpkin halves.

Stir-fry vegetables

Green is always good - just like this pan of vegetables. Especially after exercise, it offers a valuable energy kick.

ingredients

- 75 grams of leeks
- 1 half a bulb of kohlrabi
- 1 stick of celery
- 100 grams of broccoli
- 1 clove of garlic
- 1 ginger
- 1 tbsp olive oil
- 40 grams of quinoa
- 150 ml of vegetable stock
- 1 stalk of lovage
- salt
- black pepper

preparation

The leek is first cleaned, washed and cut into rings. The kohlrabi is peeled and then diced. Then the celery needs to be cut into slices. The broccoli is also washed and divided into its florets. Now the garlic has to be cut into small pieces and the ginger peeled and cut into cubes.
First, fry the garlic and ginger in a pan with heated oil. Fry the quinoa briefly. Gradually add all the vegetables and fry them for a short time. Then deglaze with the vegetable stock and let it cook for a quarter of an hour on low heat. The lovage is now cut into small strips and mixed with the food. At the end everything is seasoned as you like.

Avocado - potato salad

Potato salad is actually pretty greasy and not exactly healthy. But this variant with avocado is healthy, alkaline and delicious.

ingredients

- 1 kilogram of potatoes
- sea salt
- 2 avocados
- Lime juice
- 1 half bunch of spring onions
- 50 grams of dried tomatoes
- cress
- 1 tbsp olive oil
- 100 ml vegetable stock
- pepper
- salt
- 30 grams of pine nuts

preparation

First, the potatoes must be cleaned thoroughly - preferably with a brush or a special glove. Then they are cooked for a quarter of an hour. While the potatoes are cooling, the avocados are peeled off and cut into small pieces. Then drip lime juice over it.
Now the spring onions need to be chopped into small pieces. Then drain the tomatoes and collect the oil. Now also cut into small pieces. Put everything in a bowl and cut the cress.
Mix the oil and the stock and add to the salad. Now season everything with salt and pepper. In addition, fry the pine nuts in a pan and sprinkle over the finished salad when serving.

As you can see, there is exactly the right dish at any time of the day - and everything is tailored to the alkaline diet. But every now and then everybody gets a little hungry in between and you want to treat yourself to a small snack. Unfortunately, sugar is taboo.

What now?

Fortunately, there are enough tasty alternatives in the alkaline diet that are also ideal for a short break. Made entirely from fresh ingredients.

Ideal for in between - 4 basic snack recipes

Basic chocolate mousse

Sounds like a calorie bomb - but it's not. This dish is quick and easy. It also works completely without cream and sugar.

ingredients

- 4 bananas
- 1 avocado
- 4 dates
- 4 tbsp cocoa powder

preparation

Firstly, cut the bananas and dates into small pieces.
Then puree all the ingredients in a blender.
Fill everything into glasses and add half a date for decoration. Now sprinkle with cocoa powder.

Vegetable chips

Potato chips have not been the trend for a long time. Now come the healthy vegetable chips made from carrot and beetroot. Hardly any fat, but plenty of flavor.

ingredients

- 2 carrots
- Beetroot
- 2 teaspoons of olive oil
- 1 half teaspoon of curry powder
- 1 teaspoon of rosemary
- sea salt

preparation

First, preheat the oven to 190 degrees. Now peel the carrot and beetroot and then cut into thin slices. Let the liquid soak up with a kitchen towel.
Now put the carrots together with the olive oil and curry powder in a bowl and mix. Take another bowl and mix the beetroot, oil and rosemary in it. Then spread the vegetables on a baking sheet. Now add a generous pinch of sea salt on top.
Bake everything for about half an hour - then the vegetables are also crispy. If too much steam is generated, the oven should be opened from time to time.
When preparing it, make sure that all the chips are of the same thickness otherwise they will quickly turn black. By the way, you can also use other types of vegetables.

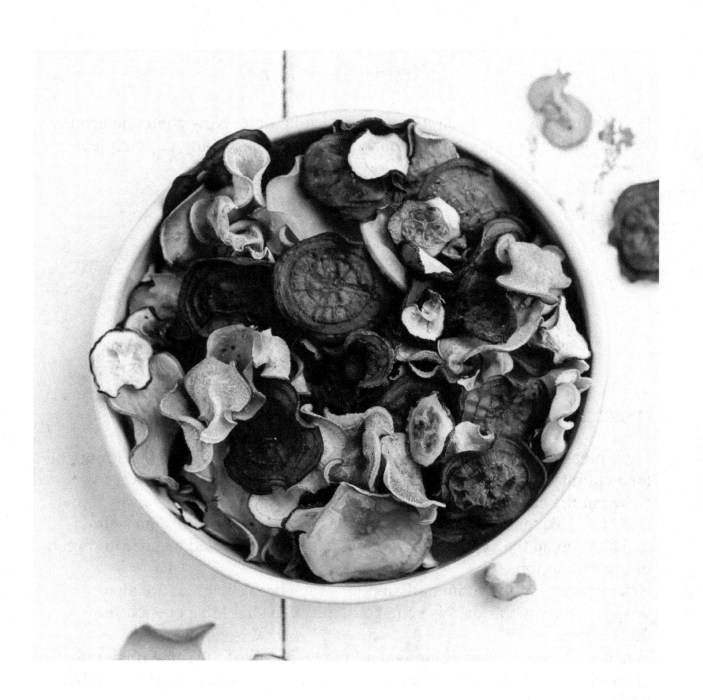

Beetroot cream

A dry side dish goes best with this dish, because this cream has a very intense taste.

ingredients

- 2 scoops of beetroot
- 100 grams of chickpeas
- 2 teaspoons of dill
- 1 half teaspoon coriander
- 1 teaspoon lemon juice
- sea salt
- black pepper

preparation

Boil the beetroot in salted water for half an hour. When it has cooled down, peel and cut into pieces.
Now add the lemon juice, the chickpeas and the spices and puree everything in the blender. Now season with sea salt and pepper.

Cashew spread

This spread is ideal for small hunger pangs. With its nutty note, it still has a fruity aftertaste.

ingredients

- 2 handfuls of cashew nuts
- 2 shallots
- 1 clove of garlic
- 1 ginger
- 2 tbsp rapeseed oil
- 2 carrots
- 2 apples
- 5 stalks of thyme
- 1 tbsp agave syrup
- lemon juice
- salt
- pepper

preparation

The kernels must be roughly chopped and then roasted in a pan over medium heat. They need to tan easily. Then shallots, garlic and also ginger are peeled and chopped into small cubes. Then fry with rapeseed oil.
Now peel and grate the carrot. Remove the seeds from the apples and cut into cubes. Put the carrots in the pan and fry for a short time. Finally, apple and thyme are added. Then put the mixture with the cashews in a container and puree with a hand blender.
Finally, add salt and pepper as desired and store in glasses with screw caps in the refrigerator.

That was a lot of choice of recipes for every occasion. However, if you want to take an intensive cure with an alkaline diet, you need a lot more. After all, there should be no boredom.

Therefore, here are more basic diet recipes for guaranteed every occasion - healthy and with a guaranteed taste!

Always ready - 43 other basic recipes ideal for basic cures

Special kale salad

Green food is all the rage right now. Of course - it's not only healthy, but also looks great.

ingredients

- 250 grams of kale
- 200 grams of edamame
- 75 grams of cranberries
- 10 cherry tomatoes
- 4 tablespoons of olive oil
- lemon juice
- salt

preparation

Remove the stalk from the kale, wash it off, and then dry it off. It is then placed in a bowl and cut into small pieces. Now we mix the olive oil with the salt and lemon juice. This dressing is then kneaded into the salad for a few minutes. Then put the whole thing in the refrigerator for a short time. During this time you can put the edamame in boiling salted water and let it cook for around four minutes. Then drain and cool briefly. Now the tomatoes are washed and divided in half.
Now add the tomatoes, edamame and cranberries to the kale and season to taste.

Curry pan with potatoes

A curry is not only fancy and spicy, but can also achieve an optimal alkaline effect with the right vegetables.

ingredients

- 400 grams of potatoes
- 1 pointed cabbage
- 1 bell pepper
- 2 carrots
- 2 tablespoons of oil
- 2 onions
- 2 teaspoons of turmeric
- 1 teaspoon of curry
- 1 half can of coconut milk
- salt
- pepper
- 2 tbsp sesame seeds

preparation

The pointed cabbage needs to be washed. Then the stalk is removed, the cabbage is divided into four parts and finally cut into small strips. Then the onions are peeled and diced. The peppers have to be washed and also cut into strips.

Now you can heat oil in a pan and fry onions, carrots and potatoes in it for about 10 minutes. The pointed cabbage is also fried for three minutes. The whole thing is steamed until the pointed cabbage is soft.

You can now add the spices and coconut milk and let everything boil again. The curry is now sprinkled with sesame seeds when serving.

Almond milk shake

Almond milk is a very tasty alternative to conventional milk. It is particularly good that the small nut also fits perfectly into an alkaline diet.

ingredients

- 500 ml almond milk
- 2 bananas
- 3 tbsp almond butter
- 4 ice cubes

preparation

First, the bananas need to be peeled. Now the almond milk, the puree and the ice cubes are put into a very strong mixer and pureed. After a minute of mixing, it becomes an almond milk shake.
Then put in a cool place.

Potato dumplings

These dumplings not only have a basic effect, but are also a suitable recipe if you want to shed a few pounds.

ingredients

- 6 potatoes
- parsley
- 2 teaspoons of olive oil
- herbal salt
- white pepper
- Nutmeg

preparation

The first thing to do is to peel the potatoes and cut them into pieces. Then put them in the steamer for about 20 minutes - until they are tender. Meanwhile, the parsley is washed off, dried and finely chopped. Later you use part of it for garnishing.

The boiled potatoes are now processed into a pulp. This works best with a potato masher. Now you add parsley and the spices and taste the whole thing.

The mass is now formed into dumplings with two spoons, then served on a plate and garnished.

Steamed vegetables go well with this.

kohlrabi soup

Kohlrabi supports the stomach and intestines - it also has an alkaline effect. Selenium and vitamins can even help prevent cancer.

ingredients

- 5 kohlrabi
- 2 potatoes
- 1 shallot
- 3 tablespoons of oil
- 750 ml of water
- vegetable broth
- herbal salt
- Nutmeg
- white pepper
- Allspice
- parsley

preparation

The potatoes and kohlrabi need to be washed. Then they are peeled and cut into large pieces. The shallot also needs to be peeled and finely chopped. The oil is heated and the shallot is fried for about 2 minutes. Now kohlrabi and potatoes are added and the whole thing is briefly steamed. Then you fill up the water with the broth and bring the soup to a boil. Now cook for a quarter of an hour.
Now the spices are added and the whole soup is pureed with a stick. In the meantime, wash and chop the parsley. This is then added when serving. It is particularly healthy that the soup is prepared without cream.

The special dressing

A healthy dressing is always a good addition to a refreshing salad.

ingredients

- 3 tbsp orange juice
- 1 tbsp lemon juice
- 3 tbsp sesame tahini
- 1 tbsp olive oil
- 1 tbsp maple syrup
- salt
- black pepper

preparation

To make the dressing, orange and lemon are first freshly squeezed.
Then measure the exact amount and mix everything well with the tahini,
oil, maple syrup, salt and pepper.
Then you can add it very well to a leaf or broccoli salad.

Mediterranean vegetables from the oven

ingredients

- 2 zucchinis
- 3 peppers
- 10 cherry tomatoes
- 1 half eggplant
- 1 onion
- black olives
- 1 clove of garlic
- Thyme
- Oregano
- basil
- black pepper
- 4 tablespoons of olive oil

preparation

First, all the vegetables are washed. The peppers are pitted and cut into small pieces. Eggplant and zucchini are cut into slices. After the onions and the garlic have been peeled, you can also chop them up. Now the herbs are washed off and cut. The olives are also cut up. The tomatoes, on the other hand, remain whole.
Now everything comes in a large baking dish and then the herbs on top. Add plenty of olive oil.
The vegetables are now cooked in a preheated oven at 180 degrees for half an hour. Then add salt and pepper.

Eggplant rolls with basil

This dish is a real delicacy when warm, but can also be eaten cold as a snack in between.It is delicious in all variations.

ingredients

- 1 eggplant
- 2 tablespoons of olive oil
- 4 potatoes
- basil
- herbal salt
- white pepper

preparation

First, the eggplants are washed and cleaned. Then they are cut into very thin slices and sprinkled with salt. Let the whole thing stand for about 20 minutes.
In addition, the potatoes are peeled and cut into cubes. They are then immersed in boiling salted water for just under half an hour. Alternatively, you can also use a steamer.
The eggplants are meanwhile coated with oil and grilled in the oven.
The basil is washed off and also cut into small pieces.
When the potatoes are ready, they are mashed and mixed with the oil, salt, pepper and the basil. If necessary, you can also add a little water.
The mass is now formed into small dumplings, which are then wrapped with the eggplant slices. A wooden skewer is used to ensure that everything stays in place.

KiBa - smoothie

ingredients

- 500 grams of cherries
- 1 banana
- 5 lemon balm leaves

preparation

All cherries are pitted and washed. The banana is peeled and cut into large pieces.
Both go into the mixer and are pureed. If necessary, you can also add water.
When the smoothie is ready, it is filled into glasses and decorated with lemon balm.

Basic dressing

A basic dressing is really suitable for every salad.

ingredients

- lemon
- 4 tablespoons of olive oil
- 2 tbsp parsley
- black pepper
- herbal salt

preparation

First, the lemon is squeezed out and mixed with the olive oil in a bowl. Meanwhile, the parsley and the other herbs are made small and simply lifted under the now finished dressing.

Soup made from nettles

Nettle - a common natural remedy for many years.

ingredients

- 180 grams of nettles
- 4 potatoes
- 1 onion
- 6 tablespoons of olive oil
- 500 ml of vegetable stock
- 300 ml of water
- Nutmeg
- salt
- pepper
- 2 tbsp sesame seeds

preparation

For the soup you first have to remove the skin from the onion and cut it into small pieces. Then it is fried in hot olive oil.
Now the leaves of the nettle need to be plucked, washed and steamed in a saucepan until they disintegrate.
You can also add the potatoes - peeled and cut into cubes. Now the vegetable broth is topped up and the whole thing has to cook for half an hour. Now it has to be mashed. In the meantime, the sesame is briefly toasted.
The soup is now seasoned with the various spices and served. Sprinkle with the sesame seeds. But you can also leave them out.

Chili pumpkin

ingredients

- 1 Hokkaido pumpkin
- 3 chili peppers
- 1 tbsp honey
- 4 tablespoons of lemon juice
- Coriander
- 6 tablespoons of olive oil
- salt
- black pepper

preparation

First of all, the pumpkin is washed and put in the oven completely, baked for 20 minutes at 150 degrees. So it can be cut better. After it has cooled, it is cut in half and the kernels and stalk are removed. Now you can cut it into slices - but the pumpkin doesn't have to be peeled.

Then the chili peppers are cleaned, pitted and chopped up into small pieces. The small pieces are mixed together with olive oil, honey, coriander and lemon juice.

During this time, the pumpkin is placed on a new tray and coated with the marinade. When the oven is preheated, everything will cook for about 20 minutes.

Then it is seasoned with pepper and salt and then served.

Turmeric smoothie

ingredients

- 60 grams of spinach leaves
- 1 banana
- 200 ml of water
- 2 tbsp almond butter
- 1 tbsp linseed oil
- cinnamon
- turmeric

preparation

The spinach leaves are washed and put in the blender. Then add the puree, the banana, water, cinnamon and turmeric. Everything is pureed into a creamy smoothie.

Millet porridge

Doesn't sound very tasty and exciting - but it is.

ingredients

- 400 grams of pumpkin
- 200 grams of potatoes
- 150 grams of millet
- 400 ml of water
- 1.5 apples
- 100 ml apple juice
- 1 tbsp rapeseed oil

preparation

The potatoes and pumpkin are washed, peeled and cut into cubes. Then put the millet with both and the water in a saucepan and cook it over medium heat for a quarter of an hour.

Now the apples can also be washed, peeled and their pits removed. Then they are cut into cubes and placed in the saucepan for 5 minutes. Don't forget to stir, because the dish can burn very easily.

Now you take the pot off the stove and add the apple juice. Now puree everything as you like. You can also add water for dilution. Mix in the rapeseed oil when serving.

You can also freeze this food.

Millet porridge

Porridge is full of healthy ingredients and is ideal for an alkaline breakfast every day.

ingredients

- 120 grams of millet
- 200 ml of water
- 150 ml of water
- 125 grams of apple
- 4 dried apricots
- cinnamon
- 2 tbsp coconut flakes
- 1 tbsp sesame seeds
- 2 tablespoons of flaxseed

preparation

First, the millet must be rinsed off thoroughly and cooked in a saucepan with the flax seeds, sesame seeds, water and coconut milk.
Now the apple is washed, the stones removed and cut into pieces. Now put in the pot and cook with it. Cut the apricots and add them. Leave on the stove for 5 minutes and then swell at half heat.
If necessary, a little coconut milk can be mixed in, as well as the cinnamon and the roasted coconut flakes.

Basic breakfast cereal

This alkaline food can be prepared very well in advance - without the fresh fruit - and stored for several weeks.

ingredients

- 20 grams of millet
- 50 grams of buckwheat
- 30 grams of pumpkin seeds
- 30 grams of sunflower seeds
- 3 dates
- 1 apple
- cinnamon
- 400 ml of water

preparation

The millet, buckwheat, seeds and nuts are made small with a suitable mixer. Now cut the fig and also the dates into very small pieces. Put everything together in a saucepan and bring to the boil with the water. Then cook on low heat for 3 minutes.
Meanwhile you can wash and peel the apple. Cut into small pieces.
The basic muesli now has to cool down and mixed with apple and cinnamon. Finally the muesli can be served.

Purslane salad

Tip - grapeseed oil is the perfect substitute for conventional oils.

ingredients

- 200 grams of purslane
- 250 grams of cherry tomatoes
- 200 grams of chanterelles
- 2 tbsp rapeseed oil
- 2 tablespoons of linseed oil
- 2 tablespoons of vinegar
- 30 ml of orange juice
- salt
- black pepper
- garlic

preparation

First of all, you need to wash the tomatoes and cut them in half. Now wash the mushrooms briefly and check for spots. Very small mushrooms can be processed in this way, otherwise cut into large slices. Wash the leaves of the purslane and put everything in a large bowl.
Now the garlic is peeled and pressed. Then mix with the vinegar and the spices. Mix with the oils to make a vinaigrette. Now the salad can be dressed with the dressing and served.

Thai quinoa salad

ingredients

- 200 grams of quinoa
- 400 ml of water
- 1 bell pepper
- 1 carrot
- 1 cucumber
- 2 spring onions
- Coriander
- 3 limes
- 2 tbsp fish sauce
- 3 tablespoons of olive oil
- 2 tablespoons of sugar
- 2 chili peppers
- salt

preparation

Quinoa is rinsed well through a sieve and then steamed with a little oil. Then the water is poured on and everything is boiled with a little salt. Then continue to simmer over low heat - until there is no more water. Let cool and then loosen up.

Make a salad dressing from the fish sauce, the juice, sugar, olive oil and the chopped chili peppers. It works well if you shake all the ingredients in a sealed glass. How many chili peppers you use depends on personal taste. You can of course leave them out entirely.

Peel the cucumber and dice with paprika. The spring onions are cut into small pieces and everything is added to the dressing with the chopped coriander. Now that comes to the salad. At the end it is still seasoned.

Buckwheat porridge

ingredients

- 2 apples
- 2 carrots
- 1 banana
- 50 grams of buckwheat semolina
- 400 ml of water
- 1 tbsp rapeseed oil
- 3 tbsp walnuts
- salt

preparation

The first thing to do is to boil the water with the salt. The buckwheat semolina is then washed with hot water. Now you can take the pot off and add the semolina. Let simmer for five minutes on a low heat - but don't forget to stir.

During this time you can wash, peel and grate the apple and carrots. The banana is mashed. Now everything can be pureed together with a little oil. Stir the fruit and carrots into the warm porridge and pour into small bowls.

Fennel soup with zucchini

ingredients

- 2 bulbs of fennel
- 2 zucchinis
- 80 grams of onion
- 1 tbsp butter
- white pepper
- 500 ml of vegetable stock
- salt

preparation

The fennel is washed and the stalk is removed. The green can be kept for decoration. Now the fennel is cut into cubes.

Remove the skin from the zucchini and cut into small slices. The onion is also chopped.

Now the butter is made hot in a saucepan and the fennel and zucchini are steamed for 3 minutes.

Top up with vegetable stock and cook everything for about a quarter of an hour over a very low flame. Then the fennel should be soft.

The soup is now pureed and, if necessary, a little more water is added. Now it is seasoned with salt and pepper.

At the end, the green from the fennel is finely chopped and added to the soup served in a plate.

Broccoli Salad with Quinoa

ingredients

- 100 grams of quinoa
- 1 broccoli
- 300 ml vegetable stock
- 25 ml of lemon juice
- 4 tablespoons of olive oil
- black pepper
- salt
- parsley
- 80 grams of onions
- 1 clove of garlic

preparation

First, the quinoa is rinsed in a colander under cold water and then brought to the boil in a saucepan with the vegetable stock. After ten minutes, drain again in a colander
The lemon is squeezed out for the dressing. Now the parsley is washed and dried again. The clove of garlic and the onions are peeled off and finely chopped with the parsley. The ingredients are now mixed into the dressing and seasoned with salt and pepper.
Now the broccoli is washed and the small roses are separated. You have to chop it up and add it to the quinoa. Now the dressing is added and the salad is served in a bowl.

Vegetables from the oven

ingredients

- 2 zucchinis
- 4 potatoes
- 10 cherry tomatoes
- 3 carrots
- Thyme
- rosemary
- parsley
- black pepper
- salt
- 4 tablespoons of olive oil

preparation

The vegetables are washed off, and potatoes and carrots are peeled and cut into small pieces. The zucchinis are cut into slices. Only the tomatoes remain whole.

Now everything comes in a very large baking dish. Add the herbs and plenty of olive oil to mix.

If the oven is preheated, everything is baked at 180 degrees for half an hour. Every now and then you should stir and possibly add some water. When the vegetables are ready, add salt and pepper to taste and then serve.

Quinoa and carrot salad

ingredients

- 200 grams of quinoa
- 5 carrots
- 100 grams of almonds
- 1 lemon
- 1 clove of garlic
- parsley
- 3 tbsp sesame tahini
- 4 tablespoons of olive oil
- 50 grams of raisins

preparation

The quinoa is washed in a sieve under running water and then cooked in salted water for twenty minutes.

The carrots also have to be washed, then peeled and cut into wafer-thin slices.

Now wash the parsley, pluck it and coarsely chop it together with the almonds. Now wash the lemon and rub off half of the peel. The lemon is halved and all the juice is squeezed out. Remove the garlic from the skin and chop it very finely.

The garlic and the grated peel are now mixed with the tahini, spices and lemon juice. The oil is also added.

At the end everything is mixed together and has to be steeped briefly.

Carrot Millet Bread

This gluten-free bread is a great alternative to normal bread.

ingredients

- 150 grams of buckwheat
- 200 grams of millet
- 200 grams of carrots
- 125 grams of oatmeal
- 550 ml of water
- 2 teaspoons of salt
- 50 grams of sunflower seeds
- 25 grams of flaxseed oil
- 25 grams of sesame seeds
- 30 grams of psyllium husks
- 1 pack of gluten-free baking powder
- 3 tablespoons of olive oil

preparation

The carrots are roughly chopped and mashed with a blender. But you can also rub them.

Buckwheat and millet are also crushed in a blender so that they become flour.

The dry ingredients are now mixed together and processed into a bread dough with the carrots and water. But you shouldn't add all of the water immediately and the dough should neither be too soft nor too firm.

Now you have to line a loaf pan with baking paper. The bottom is sprinkled with oatmeal, and finally the dough comes in. The top of the bread must now be scratched several times with a knife.

After the oven has been preheated, the bread is baked at 200 degrees for 40 minutes. Then draw the crack and bake again for half an hour at 180 degrees. Once this has happened, the mold is taken out of the oven and has to cool down. Then cut.

You can cut a good 30 slices from such bread.

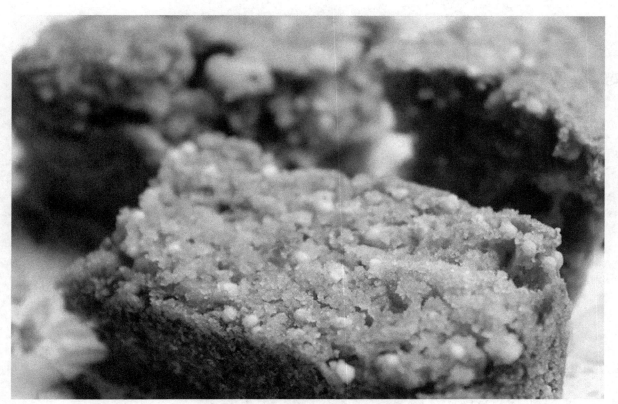

Basic stuffed peppers

ingredients

- 250 grams of quinoa
- 500 ml of vegetable stock
- 4 red peppers
- Coriander
- 2 tablespoons of olive oil
- 1 onion
- 150 ml of vegetable stock
- 80 grams of butter
- 1 teaspoon paprika powder
- black pepper

preparation

First, rinse the quinoa under warm water and bring the vegetable stock to a boil. Cook quinoa in it for half an hour over low heat.

The peppers are washed, the lid is removed and the skin and seeds are removed. The coriander must also be peeled and chopped into small pieces. Now you can coat a large baking dish with a little oil. At the same time, remove the skin from the onions and chop them into small pieces. Quinoa comes from the stove. If necessary, add a little water. In the meantime, the oven is preheated to 220 degrees.

A little oil is made hot in the pan and the onions are fried in it until translucent. Quinoa and coriander are added. The peppers are then filled with this mixture. The lid comes back on.

The peppers are now placed in the baking dish and the broth comes on the bottom. Cook the whole thing for 25 minutes at 220 degrees.

You can also melt the butter in a saucepan and season with paprika and pepper. Then serve the finished paprika and garnish with the butter.

Vegan couscous salad

ingredients

- 150 grams of couscous
- 300 ml vegetable stock
- 2 beefsteak tomatoes
- 1 bulb of fennel
- 120 grams of sugar snap peas
- 2 tbsp ajvar
- 3 tablespoons of fruit vinegar
- 180 ml of tomato juice
- 4 tablespoons of olive oil
- cress
- 160 grams of lettuce
- pepper
- salt

preparation

The cooked broth is poured over the couscous and it must soak for about 10 minutes.

The tomatoes are cut into small wedges. The fennel and the sugar snap peas, however, in fine strips. The lettuce is simply cut up and placed on four different plates.

Now the tomato juice is mixed with the ajvar, the vinegar and the olive oil. The resulting dressing is seasoned with salt and pepper.

Now add the vegetables and the sugar snap peas and everything is mixed well. Place on the plate with the lettuce and garnish with the cress at the end.

Corn salad smoothie

Lamb's lettuce is not just a popular vegetable for a crunchy smoothie. No -
it can also be used to make delicious green smoothies.

ingredients

- 125 grams of lamb's lettuce
- 1.5 bananas
- lemon juice
- 20 grams of walnuts
- 10 grams of flaxseed
- 3 tbsp sesame seeds
- 150 ml apple juice
- 250 ml of water

preparation

First of all, the lamb's lettuce must be washed. Then put it in the blender
with the banana, walnuts, lemon juice, sesame seeds, apple juice and water.
Everything is then mashed for about a minute.
This smoothie is very thick, but enough for two full glasses. It should also
be served with a spoon. With the amount of water you should proceed
according to your own gut feeling, because everyone likes it differently. Of
course, you can also add less apple juice, then the smoothie will not taste as
sweet.

Tomato broth

This recipe is not only basic, but is also based on a therapeutic fasting plan.

ingredients

- 500 grams of tomatoes
- Leeks
- Celery
- 1 carrot
- 1 teaspoon vegetable stock
- sea salt
- Nutmeg
- Oregano
- 4 teaspoons of yeast flakes

preparation

The tomatoes are washed and cut in half. The celery, carrots and leeks are also washed off and the skin removed. Then you cut everything into small cubes.

Bring one liter of water to the boil and add the vegetable stock. Cook the ingredients in it for around 20 minutes until soft.

Now the soup has to pass through a sieve. When serving, you add the yeast flakes, which you should not cook under any circumstances, otherwise vitamins and valuable folic acid will be lost.

The recipe is very good for four people.

Beetroot smoothie

This smoothie is a beginner's smoothie. Why? It actually contains a lot of vegetables, but it tastes sweet and pleasant. This smoothie is a change from the many green smoothies.

ingredients

- 1 beetroot
- 100 grams of cucumber
- 40 grams of spinach leaves
- 1 apple
- 1 orange
- 20 grams of almonds
- 15 grams of flaxseed
- 15 grams of walnuts
- 300 ml of water

preparation

The beetroot is first peeled, quartered and finally put in a normal mixer. Cucumber and apple are also washed off and chopped into pieces. They can also be peeled off if you like. You can also use a knife for the orange. Then cut it in half and put it in the blender with the almonds, flax seeds and nuts. Now puree everything for a minute.

The smoothie is good enough for three glasses. Its consistency is rather thick and should therefore be enjoyed with a spoon. If you want the smoothie to be more liquid, you should vary the amount of water.

Vegan raw vegetables salad

ingredients

- 500 grams of broccoli
- 150 grams of apple
- 1 bell pepper
- 40 grams of sunflower seeds
- olive oil
- 2 tbsp verjuice
- 1 tbsp sugar beet syrup
- salt
- pepper

preparation

The broccoli, apple and peppers are first washed off and the seeds removed. Now everything is cut into very small pieces.
To make the dressing, mix the oil, verjuice, syrup, mustard, salt and pepper together. Now add the sunflower seeds. When everything is well mixed, the salad has to steep for about a quarter of an hour.

Sweet Potato Burger

A great alternative to a traditional beef burger.

ingredients

- 2 sweet potatoes
- 1 can of kidney beans
- 60 grams of lentils
- 2 onions
- 3 tbsp corn flour
- 2 teaspoons of carob seed oil
- 1 tbsp lemon peel
- 1 teaspoon coriander
- 1 teaspoon of caraway seeds
- paprika powder
- Nutmeg
- 1 teaspoon fennel seed powder
- anise
- black pepper
- salt
- Thyme
- 4 tbsp sunflower oil
- 500 grams of sauerkraut

preparation

The sweet potatoes are steamed or alternatively cooked in the oven. Then you have to peel them. The lentils are boiled for ten minutes and then drained. Now the kidney beans are washed in a sieve and dried on kitchen paper.
The onions are peeled off and chopped into small pieces. The leaves of the thyme are plucked and also chopped up.
Now put the sweet potatoes, lentils, beans, corn flour, lemon peel, flour and all the spices together in a blender and briefly pureed - until they are

lumpy. If everything is too fine, the dough will later have the wrong consistency. Then it is seasoned with pepper and salt.

Rub your hands with corn flour and form 2 centimeters thick burgers from the mixture. This amount can be made up to eight pieces.

Fry the burgers in hot oil for three minutes on each side. Store the burgers that are already done in the warm oven.

Now heat the sauerkraut in a saucepan and serve on a plate with the burgers.

Watermelon salad

ingredients

- 350 grams of spinach leaves
- 175 grams of watermelon
- 3 tbsp sunflower seeds
- 3 tbsp sesame seeds
- 2 tbsp lime juice
- 3 tablespoons of olive oil
- 1 teaspoon maple syrup
- pepper
- salt

preparation

Firstly, you have to wash the lettuce and tear it into small pieces and cut the melon into cubes. Lime juice, sunflower seeds, sesame seeds and oil are now mixed with the maple syrup to make a dressing and seasoned with salt and pepper.
Now the salad, melon and dressing are mixed together and served on a plate or in a bowl.

Millet soy porridge

The taste of this porridge is very reminiscent of rice pudding, but it is a healthy alternative to the sweet dish. In terms of content, it scores the most with its vitamin C. It tastes delicious even without fruit and the sugar beet syrup gives the porridge that certain external something.

ingredients

- 120 grams of millet
- 280 ml soy milk

- 20 grams of sugar beet syrup
- 1 tbsp almond butter
- lemon juice
- 40 grams of raspberries
- salt

preparation

The millet is washed with hot water and then boiled in the soy milk for about five minutes.
Then add the almond butter, the syrup, the lemon juice and a little salt. Now the whole thing has to swell again for 10 minutes.

Salad smoothie

ingredients

- 1 orange
- 1 apple
- 1 half avocado
- 1 cucumber
- 100 grams of spinach leaves
- parsley
- 100 grams of lamb's lettuce
- 2 tbsp sunflower seeds
- 2 tablespoons of flaxseed
- 150 ml of water

preparation

Flax seeds and the sunflower seeds must first swell together in a cup with a little water.

In the meantime, the avocado can be peeled. Cucumber, parsley and lettuce are washed and then everything goes into the blender.

Now peel the orange with a knife and cut it in half or third. The apples are also washed, pitted and cut into small pieces.

Everything goes into a stand mixer and is pureed for about a minute.

With this amount of ingredients, you get about three glasses full. This smoothie should also be consumed with a spoon, because it is also quite thick. Of course, water can also be added and apple juice reduced. Whatever you want.

Strawberry fruit salad

A breakfast made from pure basic ingredients.

ingredients

- 2 apples
- 250 grams of strawberries
- 80 grams of blueberries
- 2 kiwis
- 150 ml of orange juice
- 1 orange
- 200 grams of tiger nuts flakes

preparation

The peel is removed from the apples and then processed into puree using a grater. The rest of the fruit is also cut into small pieces. Everything comes in one large bowl.
Now the orange juice has to be mixed with the tiger nut flakes. It has to swell for a moment and then everything can be mixed up.

Ratatouille

The French national dish is with a difference.

ingredients

- 1 eggplant
- 3 tomatoes
- 1 zucchini
- 150 ml of vegetable stock
- 3 tablespoons of olive oil
- sea salt
- Thyme
- 1 onion

preparation

The eggplant and zucchini are cut into small pieces. Boiling water is poured over the tomatoes and then left to stand. Finally, you can peel off the skin and divide it into eight equal parts.

Cut the onion into small pieces and sauté in a little hot olive oil. Then add the zucchini and eggplant and both are steamed. Top up the vegetable stock and add the tomatoes. Season everything with salt and the herbs and finally serve after a cooking time of ten minutes.

Tip - you should always use sea salt for an alkaline treatment.

Sprouts-carrots

ingredients

- 5 carrots
- 15 grams of Provence herbs
- 2 tablespoons of olive oil
- black pepper
- 1 teaspoon sunflower seeds
- 20 ml of lemon juice
- 1 onion
- 2 tbsp bean sprouts

preparation

First, mix the dressing with the olive oil, lemon juice, some salt and herbs. Then the carrots are washed and grated with a grater. The onion is peeled off and finely chopped. Everything is mixed up and the bean sprouts are added. If you like, you can sprinkle a few sunflower seeds on top.

Tomato with zucchini

Both types of vegetables are surprisingly low in carbohydrates and are also suitable for the low-carb diet.

ingredients

- 4 tomatoes
- 2 zucchinis
- 2 spring onions
- 10 black olives
- 3 tablespoons of olive oil
- 1 teaspoon herbs of Provence
- salt

preparation

You have to wash the zucchinis and then cut them into thin slices. The spring onions are cut into rings. Everything is now steamed in hot olive oil. Now the olives have to lose their stone. The tomatoes are washed and divided into eight parts. Both go into the pan.
The herbs can be added as desired and the whole thing is briefly seared and can finally be served.

Potatoes with avocado cream

ingredients

- 1 avocado
- 6 potatoes
- lemon juice
- pepper
- salt

preparation

The potatoes have to cook in hot, salted water for about 20 minutes until they are cooked through.
The avocado is divided and the core is removed. Put some lemon juice into the meat and mash it with a fork. Season to taste with salt and pepper and then simply serve with the potatoes. You can also use different herbs for decoration.
The few ingredients make this dish perfect for an alkaline treatment.

Parsnip soup

ingredients

- 3 parsnips
- 1 liter of vegetable stock
- salt
- 50 grams of celery
- 1 can of tomatoes
- 1 onion
- 1 bay leaf
- parsley

preparation

Firstly, the parsnips are cleaned and then cut into small pieces.
Celery and the onion also need to be cut into small cubes. The prepared
vegetables are now in the broth and have to cook briefly, finally a bay leaf
is added and everything cooks for another half an hour.
When it's over, add the tomatoes and cook for another 10 minutes.
Then you can remove the bay leaf again and puree the whole soup.
Now the spices are added depending on the taste - that can also be a little
more. Completely different spices are of course also allowed.

Broccoli cream soup

ingredients

- 500 grams of broccoli
- 700 grams of potatoes
- 2 onions
- 80 grams of cream
- Nutmeg
- 3 tablespoons of olive oil
- 1.5 liters of vegetable stock

preparation

The potatoes have to be peeled and washed first, the broccoli is just washed.
Then the onions and potatoes are cut into small pieces. Both come together
in a saucepan with hot oil and sauté briefly. Now the vegetable stock is
poured and everything has to simmer for a quarter of an hour.
The broccoli is made small and added. Let simmer for another three
minutes and then remove the pot from the flame. Now the soup is finely
pureed and allowed to cook for another five minutes.
At the end it is refined with the spices and the cream.

Green curry coconut soup

ingredients

- 2 avocados
- 1 half can of coconut milk
- 1 teaspoon of curry
- 600 ml of vegetable stock
- lemon juice
- salt pepper

preparation

The avocados are first pitted and peeled, then put in the blender.
The vegetable stock is added and both are mixed well.
Now add the coconut milk, curry, lemon juice, salt and pepper and puree
again until the liquid is creamy.
The soup still has to be seasoned and possibly put in the cold.

Sesame and carrot salad

ingredients

- 500 grams of carrots
- 1 apple
- ginger
- sugar
- parsley
- 1 tbsp lemon juice
- 1 tbsp apple juice
- 3 tbsp rapeseed oil
- salt
- water
- 1 tbsp sesame seeds
- pepper

preparation

The carrots are peeled off and cut into thin slices. The sugar must melt in a saucepan and then pour over the carrots.
Add the salt, some grated ginger and water and everything is steamed for about 10 minutes. At the end of the day, the carrots should still be crisp.
Now the apples are cut into small pieces and steamed briefly. Then everything has to cool down.
Now the dressing is made from lemon juice, apple juice, the spices and the oil and mixed with the salad.

The avocado

Hardly any food is more versatile and healthier than this - the
avocado. Included in many alkaline diet recipes, it has of course also
deserved its own chapter in this book.
What is the avocado all about?
And why is she so healthy?

The avocado belongs to the laurel family and is basically a fruit - actually a
berry. Many people still think it's a vegetable. Incidentally, it is also known
colloquially as butter fruit.

It naturally grows on a tree found in the tropical rainforests of Mexico and
Central America. Today there are well over 400 varieties that grow, for
example, in South Africa, California and even Spain. However, they have
only been at home there since the last century.
The avocado was already grown as a fruit by the Indian cultures in southern
Mexico 10,000 years ago. Spanish explorers first saw them in Colombia
and eventually took them to the Caribbean and South America. From there
it spread to Africa and Asia in the middle of the 19th century.
The export of avocados to the USA and finally to all of Europe began fairly
late - only after the Second World War. France, Great Britain and Germany
topped the list.
 The fruit of the avocado tree has the shape of a pear, but it can also be
round. Different species have different sizes and texture of the outer shell -
from wrinkled to smooth. The colors can also be different.
The core is quite large, located in the middle, and consists of two
halves. The flesh is usually yellowish, but can get dark in the fresh air.

The avocados are available in almost every store these days. Sometimes a
bit hard, but you can still buy them. In any case, they will still be really
ripe. If the peel is a little soft, then the perfect degree of ripeness has been
reached and you can eat it. Incidentally, no avocado is harvested from the
tree when it is ripe - they simply fall down, where they are then picked up

by the harvest workers. The most common variety is the "Fuerte". A pear-shaped avocado that is also very popular in German retail.
This fruit can also become quite large and weigh up to 2.5 kilograms. Generally, they are high in healthy fats and potassium.

The avocado is on many menus around the world - but how is it consumed now?
The peel and the huge core are not suitable for consumption, but the particularly nutritious pulp is. In some countries - for example in Mexico - the leaves of the plant are also used as a spice.
By nature, avocados don't taste sweet, but they have the highest fat content of all types of fruit. The pulp can be eaten raw - either pure or refined with lemon juice or salt.

The avocado can still be used in so many ways:

☐ Avocado **cream** - This is a **puree** made from the pulp of the avocado. In the USA and Mexico in particular, the cream is very popular as a dip, spread or filling for dishes. The preparation is relatively easy. You just have to remove the pulp and then puree in a blender. Then - depending on your personal taste - ingredients and spices are added. By the way, this cream is also called guacamole.
☐ **Sandwiches** - In Australia and New Zealand it is common to put the avocado between two slices of toast and then serve it with the chicken.
☐ **Sauce** - In Chile, for example, the avocado is made into a sauce that is spread on burgers, hot dogs or a salad.
☐ **Salad** - As a salad, the fruit is mostly eaten in African countries. But here in Europe, too, this type of preparation has become very popular in vegan and alkaline kitchens.
☐ Dessert **or alcohol** - on other parts of the world, avocados are made into desserts such as shakes. The Indians made an alcoholic drink out of the fruit.
☐ **Medicine** - Avocado can be used, for example, to treat diarrhea or for controlled weight gain . But there is also a certain healing effect for overweight people, because daily consumption is not only healthy, but also lowers cholesterol levels.

☐ **Oil -** The oil of the avocado was already used by the Aztecs. From time to time edible oil is made from it, but today it is more used in cosmetics.

Why is this particular fruit so healthy for the body?

For a long time, the avocado was just a food that made you fat. Sure, with so much fat in it. Nowadays, however, the avocado is considered a true superfood and should, if possible, be consumed every day.
But fat and superfood really don't go together. Or?
Yes, because the avocado contains a lot of healthy fats. Studies in recent years have also shown that sugar and carbohydrates are more likely to lead to long-term obesity. The avocado is not at all to blame. With it you can maintain your weight or even reduce it in the end, because these fats make you full longer.
But of course that is not the only advantage of the extraordinary fruit - there is much more to it. Lots of vitamins, cartinoids, biotin and folic acid. And these are only a few examples, because the amino acids that are important for life can also be found in it.

By the way, the healthy superfruit can do the following:

☐ Lower cholesterol levels with healthy fats. The risk of suffering a heart attack is significantly reduced.
☐ You become more beautiful with avocados. The carotenoids contained protect against harmful UV light. Vitamins stimulate the body's own production of collagen and biotin ensures strong hair and nails.
☐ The risk of developing age-related eye diseases is reduced. Above all, the carotenoids play a decisive role in the visual processes.
☐ In 2015, a substance was found in the avocado that may help heal blood cancer. Avocatin successfully fights stem cells. But this still needs some research, and the fact alone is a major breakthrough in medicine.
☐ The avocado just tastes good - aromatic and yet mild. You can prepare it in a wide variety of ways and it is also perfect for basic cuisine.

More tips on an alkaline diet

Of course, there are people who will see absolutely no point in an alkaline diet, but numerous experts have long since confirmed the assumptions - an alkaline diet is extremely healthy and can prevent many diseases.
An intensive cure is a good start, even if it's only for a few days. The focus is on a diet with alkaline foods, but other useful tips can be used to achieve the best possible effect on the body.

Here are 10 simple tips for an alkaline diet:

☐ Have **snacks** ready
Who doesn't know him? The cravings
He is particularly present in times of boredom or especially during short breaks at work. You need something between your teeth, so you often turn to unhealthy foods. But it is better if you prepare. Simply prepare a can of cut fruit and vegetables in good time. If you are now hungry, you can reach into the can without feeling guilty. It's all a matter of getting used to. Incidentally, this also works in the evening in front of the television.

☐ Plan **the purchase**
If you walk into a store haphazardly and, worst of all, hungry, you can quickly fall for the corporate marketing tricks. By the way, there are special offers especially for unhealthy foods, such as fast food or sweets. But if you put together a list of things you need for a week beforehand, you won't fall victim to these tricks so easily. In addition, you can better plan the basic recipes.

☐ Ban on **sweets**
Sugar is poison for our body, which is considered to be the most powerful acid generator. It can also lead to obesity or even an addiction. This is exactly why you should ban all sweets from the house right from the start. But if you still need something sweet every now and then to keep you happy, you are welcome to use

alternative substitutes - for example xylitol or stevia. Fruit isn't exactly bitter either.

☐ **No luxury foods**

As difficult as it is - the daily coffee at the breakfast table has to go. Just like the beer after work. After all, these are just habits that you can work off yourself. They also mess up the acid-base balance. But watch out - red wine, for example, can have an alkaline effect in certain quantities and is therefore not that unhealthy.

☐ **lemon** water

Lemons are naturally sour. However, anyone who thinks that adding lemon to water can lead to acidification is wrong. Because the metabolism ensures that this sour lemon juice is really converted into bases. And that is healthy.

☐ Consume **chlorophyll**

Chlorophyll comes from plants and is one of nature's strongest protective mechanisms. It gets into the body through green vegetables - for example spinach, broccoli or kale. There are also special dietary supplements that contain the substance.

☐ **An overview helps**

Before you start with an alkaline diet, you must of course be clear which products are alkaline and which do not. There are enough lists of them on the Internet and of course in this book. It is best to learn them by heart. It's not that easy, but it helps prevent a lack of planning when shopping.

☐ Understand **relationships**

The whole subject of alkaline nutrition is not easy to understand. But if you still want to change your lifestyle sustainably, you should read carefully beforehand.

☐ **testing**

And you can do it yourself. Special test strips for urine are available in the pharmacy. In this way you can quickly get a rough overview of the balance in the acid-base balance.

☐ Start **the cure**

If you have followed all the instructions, you can start. In the beginning, it will not be very easy to change the existing habits - especially in the first few days. Cravings can therefore be the result from the very first evening. Of course, you shouldn't give in to that, otherwise you quickly fall back into old routines. Should a mistake happen, it is no end of the world. Changing your diet takes time.

Alkaline and vegan diet

A problem often arises, especially on public holidays and birthdays - you want to conjure up a true star menu. However, vegans also sit at the table. However, if you rely on basic food, then that's not so bad at all. On the contrary, it goes perfectly together.

At the beginning, it should be said that a vegan diet is definitely not the same as an alkaline diet. However, most vegan foods are much more basic than a normal meal. This type of diet also includes a certain amount of white flour and proteins, which unfortunately can also form acids. However, this can be compensated for by the high proportion of fruit and vegetables.

For a vegan and basic menu for a party, you can suggest the following dishes:

starter
Vegetable soup or lamb's lettuce with fresh herbs

Main course
Risotto with fresh vegetables or a vegan roast with sweet potatoes

dessert
Fruit sorbet

More detailed recipes can be found earlier in this book.
In the end, a vegan and alkaline meal doesn't have to be boring and tasteless. On the contrary, it can offer a great deal of diversity. In addition, it is healthy and sustainable.

Other diets

Breathing and nutrition are two of the most important sources of energy for our body.
This is a fact that is unfortunately all too often forgotten due to a stressful everyday life. Health is very often neglected, because fast and ready-made meals are now commonplace in households. Only a few people consciously pay attention to their diet. So a correct nutritional concept is needed.

But what does correct mean in this case?
The fact is that you can't go wrong with an alkaline diet. But there are also alternatives that can also be combined quite well with the basic diet.
It is important that the diet also suits the person in question. The latest hype is not always the perfect personal solution. Incidentally, you should not only think about changing your diet when you feel the first symptoms of an illness in your body.

As an example, a diet is presented that is perfectly in harmony with the alkaline diet - the 5-element teaching of TCM.
TCM is traditional Chinese medicine and the 5-element theory is a nutritional theory that describes the "power of the middle". It is the ability to transform food and pass on the nutrients obtained from it to the whole organism.
According to the Chinese, however, this ability is weakened in Europe and America today. However, regular meals should be able to prevent this - as long as they are prepared with foods that are easily digestible. In this way the power of the center is preserved and also strengthened.
The principle is that the food you eat provides vital energy. This gives you strength for the stressful everyday life and also increases your own performance. In addition, acidification is avoided and toxic waste products cannot even arise.

There are also many similarities with the world-famous detox, i.e. detoxifying the body. Both cures can also be wonderfully combined with one another.

But what is it all about?

The term "detox" is on everyone's lips - whether among celebrities in Hollywood or in modern households around the world.

As expected, the name comes from English and means something like detoxification or purification. Strictly speaking, the term was actually used for drug withdrawal - after all, it also removes toxins from the body. It is now used in many other areas.

And that is exactly where the problem lies. The name of Detox is unfortunately not legally protected and so each provider can decide for himself what he understands by it. That doesn't always have something to do with the actual basic idea.

Detox is actually almost the same as fasting. Partly - or sometimes completely - certain foods are avoided, such as fast food or an unhealthy diet in general. Often, however, drinks, luxury foods and smoking are also taboo, because this is also how harmful substances can get into the body. Many religions and peoples practice fasting, for example Christianity or Islam. There it is a form of repentance.

In these days of cures and therapies, the detox often only serves the goal of losing weight. The thought of detoxification or purification is unfortunately often lost from sight.

The actual story behind the creation of Detox goes back a long way into the past. A certain form of purification was already used in ancient India - the Panchakarme. It was part of the popular Ayurveda.

In Europe, however, the idea of detoxification did not arrive until the late 19th century. Sewer systems emerged at the time and it was discovered that the kidneys and intestines could secrete pathogenic substances. But then the actual term "purification" did not come up, because at that time it was still used for cleaning railways.

Nowadays, detoxification, purification and detox are ubiquitous and have become a trend all over the world.

But how exactly does this modern form of purification work?

First of all, detox is actually just an acronym and stands for detoxification. There are many forms and very different variants of diets. As already mentioned - the term is unfortunately not legally protected. So the concepts of Detox are quite diverse.

There is the form of renunciation. This is very similar to traditional fasting. Products that contain sugar or fat, highly processed or animal products are avoided for the entire duration. Because they can be poison for our body and thus only stand in the way of detoxification.

Then there is a completely different form of detox. The required food is only absorbed in liquid form. This works with special juices, smoothies, teas and soups, but can also be done with normal foods - as they are in every household. The effect can then be intensified with powder or tablets for detox.

What's the point now?

Even back then, the discoverers of Detox saw a deeper meaning in detoxification. The body should be freed of all pollutants and the quality of life should be significantly improved again. For example, heavy metals, alcohol, nicotine and pesticides are broken down and excreted from the body. The positive side effect of this is that the kidneys and liver are also strengthened by Detox. They take care that toxins stay away from the inside.

The detox itself has unfortunately not been researched enough - just like its products. There are simply too few studies on this subject, but even many medical professionals swear by detox. Fasting also finds its place in many cultures.

Detox products in powder or tablet form are often based on zeolites. This is a substance that occurs naturally as well as can be produced artificially. They are crystals that are used in industry to harden water. But do not worry - they are of course not dangerous. On the contrary. They are able to bind certain heavy metals and thus help the body to excrete them. But of course, detox in its simplest form is also possible without these special helpers. The trick is simply to eat a healthy, low-polluting, high-fiber diet. One should rely on the body's own organs for detoxification - liver, kidney and stomach, for example - to support their work.

The Detox offers many advantages for the user on a healthy way of life. However, detoxification is also a change for the body and can therefore lead to small side effects for a short time.

That would be:

☐ **headache**
Headache does not arise from detoxification, but rather from withdrawal. You have to do without nicotine or coffee and so your blood pressure rises. That leads to pain in the head. A lot of exercise in the fresh air, however, compensates for this quite well.

☐ Coated **tongue and bad breath**
This is a very common side effect and is often seen on the third day of the regimen. Most of these symptoms go away on their own, otherwise just brush your teeth more often.

☐ **impurities**
These arise in response to detoxification. But ointments or masks help quite well against it.

☐ **Bad mood**
Eating less or having to do without your favorite products can sometimes cloud the mood. In this case, the only thing that helps is to distract and - if possible - create an atmosphere of well-being.

☐ **dizziness**
This can also happen as a result of withdrawal, but this phenomenon usually goes as quickly as it appeared.

☐ **cravings**
This is probably the side effect that everyone who has ever detoxified knows. If you eat less, you get hungry. It's good to distract yourself here. Sport is always a good alternative and also has a supportive effect.

When it comes to detox, people's opinions are divided. That's a fact. But even if there are many critics of this method, there are at least as many patrons. Because they have already recognized the many advantages of this form of purification.

These are the greatest benefits of detox

1. Energy

Energy is one of the biggest buzzwords when it comes to detox. Many people practice this method in order to get more of it. Actually, this increase in energy is also a logical consequence, since pollutants are replaced by energy-rich foods during the detox.
In addition, you automatically drink more and that brings more energy.

2. Reducing weight

Another reason to get started is to reduce weight. Stars in particular swear by the effects of detox as a diet. Although you sometimes eat a little more, you actually reduce calories. That comes from the healthy foods.
But be careful - in the long term, detox will not help you achieve your dream weight, because afterwards you often gain weight again. In order to avoid a yo-yo effect, you should change your diet over the long term after the cure.

3. Strengthened immune system

Harmful substances hinder the organs of the body in their important work. Detox helps you get rid of them pretty quickly. Now they can function properly again and the immune system becomes stronger.
The nutrients that get into the body during this detox - such as important vitamins - also help the immune system to strengthen itself naturally.

4. Better complexion

It is now known that Detox helps the organs to function properly again. The skin is the largest organ in the whole body and it is naturally well supported. A visit to the sauna can also contribute positively to detoxification. This causes the skin to lose even more toxins.

In the end, it looks firmer and more radiant. It is even believed that detox is said to be very effective against acne.

5. Reduced bad breath

Of course, not everyone has bad breath, but for those who unfortunately suffer from this fate, detox can be the salvation. There is a theory that most of the time bad breath occurs when the gastrointestinal tract is too poisoned. If, however, he can resume his full functionality - through the detoxification - then the bad breath will also disappear again. Unfortunately, this smell is a side effect during the purification process, but luckily it disappears quickly.

6. Think more clearly

The spiritual curtain that prevents a person from always thinking clearly is described as fog. During a detox cure, this suddenly disappears and thinking finally becomes clearer again. The reason is that unhealthy products can no longer find their way into the body and a healthy state can be built up inside.
Incidentally, a particularly large amount of sugar is harmful to clear thinking.

7. Healthy hair

The hair that can be seen on the head and the rest of the body is actually no longer alive, because it only grows inside - under the skin. Detox makes the hair grow faster there and ultimately appears smoother and healthier.

8. Lighter feeling

Everyone is familiar with the unpleasant feeling of fullness that sets in after a long and fatty meal. It is different with fruit and vegetables, because after consumption you feel more light and healthy.
Even after the cure, you should of course not eat too much at once, otherwise the body has too little time to fight the toxins itself. The whole

game would start over. Otherwise you will still feel carefree and light for a long time after using Detox properly.

9. Anti-aging

In order to feel beautiful and healthy in old age, many people fall back on expensive anti-aging products. But there is another way. In part, aging is accelerated even more by the many pollutants in the body. With the detox, however, these toxins are withdrawn and the process is slowed down again. Free radicals should also be considered. If these are not under control, aging is faster. Detox can help control these free radicals.

10. Feeling good

You feel really good. Whether during or after the detox - this feeling is probably the most important factor in such a cure.
While the ultimate goal may be to live healthier and lose some weight, you should only start for one reason - to end up feeling better and more alive. Detox increases the quality of life.

In addition to these astonishing advantages of detoxification, there are others for each person personally - for example, having discovered a new hobby for themselves. In summary, one can say that detox is a good way to significantly increase health and enjoyment of life in a timely manner. What more do you want?

So - don't wait long. Combine detox and an alkaline diet.

The basic 10 day cure

Bringing the body's acid-base balance back into the desired equilibrium - that is the goal of an alkaline treatment. Of course, it works best in the long term, but an intensive 10-day cure is also an optimal start.

Many people rely on this method and do this regimen at least once a year. Incidentally, an alkaline cure is also referred to as an alkaline fast. This is supposed to prevent a large number of diseases, including high blood pressure and rheumatism. On average, it is common to fast for about 7-10 days. However, as with normal therapeutic fasting, all stimulants are not dispensed with, but only acid-forming foods. A much more effective form of fasting.

Therapeutic fasting is about completely detoxifying the body of toxins - it does not harm the body either. In contrast, alkaline fasting protects the body from over-acidification.

The following foods are completely avoided during the 10 days:

- coffee
- alcohol
- sweets (sugar)
- white flour
- Animal products - but butter and cream may be the exception
- carbonated drinks

Sounds pretty tough - but it's actually not.

There are so many foods on this earth that can be prepared deliciously. They also pamper the taste buds. A good example would be smoothies, because they can be prepared quickly and they also taste good.

So the selection is large and you can decide what you want to eat during a cure as you wish. The main thing is to stick to the rules, show willpower and, in the end, persevere. Being able to say no is particularly important. But it will be rewarded - at the end of the treatment you will definitely feel much better.

Many people who are trained in the subject of "alkaline nutrition" extend their alkaline diets for up to three months. But as I said, at the beginning 10 days are enough - ideal as a first test.

However, a few things should be considered beforehand. Do not take the cure if one or more of the following applies:

- Illnesses have occurred
- pregnancy
- Breastfeeding
- younger than 18 years

Now we can start.

Water, herbal teas, and various kinds of fruits and vegetables should always be there. Then you have to read well and find the recipes that appeal to you. Then you go shopping - of course with a specially created list. To be on the safe side, you should always check whether the food in question is really basic.

The trick with the whole regimen is not to view different foods as forbidden, but to tell yourself that you are only going to avoid them for a while. In the end it is much easier for you and you don't have to think about it all day.

During the alkaline fasting period, you should bathe extensively 3 to 4 times - that is, for at least one hour. In this way, harmful substances are eliminated again. You should only use special basic additives for this bath.

It can be:

- Soda
- Dead Sea Salt
- silica
- Sango coral

It is best to use a massage sponge as an aid, because it is a very good way of removing dead skin and providing better care for the new one. Sometimes a sit or foot bath can help. Then you can put some common olive oil on yourself.

The most important thing is the nutrition plan for the 10 days. In addition, you should always make sure that you drink a lot. It is best to always put a glass of water where you are.

The cure plan

day 1

breakfast
freshly squeezed juice from a pear

snack
herbal tea

Having lunch
fennel soup

dinner
Carrot salad with pear juice

day 2

breakfast
freshly squeezed juice from an apple

snack
different types of fruit

Having lunch
stuffed peppers

Vespers
Smoothie

dinner
Salad of your choice

Day 3

<u>breakfast</u>
freshly squeezed juice from an orange

<u>snack</u>
herbal tea

<u>Having lunch</u>
Potatoes with avocado cream

<u>Vespers</u>
herbal tea

<u>dinner</u>
Fruit salad with fresh fruit

Day 4

<u>breakfast</u>
fresh fruit

<u>snack</u>
herbal tea

<u>Having lunch</u>
carrot salad

<u>Vespers</u>
herbal tea

<u>dinner</u>
fresh fruit

Day 5

<u>breakfast</u>
fruit salad

<u>snack</u>
freshly squeezed juice from apples

<u>Having</u> <u>lunch</u>
Tomato with zucchini

<u>Vespers</u>
herbal tea

<u>dinner</u>
Mediterranean vegetables

Day 6

<u>breakfast</u>
herbal tea

<u>snack</u>
banana

<u>Having</u> <u>lunch</u>
Parsnip soup

<u>Vespers</u>
freshly squeezed juice from an apple

<u>dinner</u>
Stir-fry vegetables

Day 7

<u>breakfast</u>

freshly squeezed juice from grapefruit

snack
herbal tea

Having lunch
Salad of your choice

Vespers
pineapple

dinner
green smoothie

Day 8

breakfast
Apple

snack
herbal tea

Having lunch
basic curry

Vespers
herbal tea

dinner
fruit salad

Day 9

breakfast
freshly squeezed juice from orange

<u>snack</u>
pear

<u>Having</u> <u>lunch</u>
Pumpkin out of the oven

<u>Vespers</u>
herbal tea

<u>dinner</u>
kohlrabi soup

Day 10

<u>breakfast</u>
freshly squeezed juice from a banana

<u>snack</u>
herbal tea

<u>Having</u> <u>lunch</u>
Couscous Salad

<u>Vespers</u>
Smoothie of your choice

<u>dinner</u>
fresh fruit

After these 10 days, you will almost certainly feel a lot better. You feel fit
and healthy - problems with your circulatory system can also disappear.
By the way, during the entire time it is not wrong to be active. This does not
mean overexertion, but a short walk can additionally strengthen the effect of
the alkaline treatment.

Avoid these mistakes

The decision to opt for an alkaline diet is the first step on the way to a better life. Your health and general well-being will improve significantly. However, in order for everything to go as expected, good preparation is a must.

The following mistakes should therefore be avoided at all costs:

1. Coffee withdrawal

If you plan an intensive cure of around 10 days, the preparation begins a few days in advance. From then on you should do without the routine coffee in the morning. It has a strong influence on the blood vessels. Of course, this disappears during the alkaline diet. The cycle will not cope with this right away. Headaches and dizziness can occur very easily. So you should only start with the alkaline diet when the withdrawal is over.

2. Full bowel

Many people are very reluctant to talk about the topic, and it is particularly important. People should clean the colon in advance. Complications often arise during a regimen if it has not been carried out. There are always residues in the intestine that will not be released even after a few days of alkaline nutrition. In connection with alkaline foods, they can even lead to flatulence. So it is best to cleanse the bowel every two to three days with an enema.

3. Forget to drink

Regular drinking and eating are very important for our body, especially during an intensive cure with an alkaline diet. This is because around 2.5 liters of fluid are required per day. Internal organs and connective tissue are washed around and freed from harmful substances. However, you should use pure spring water, because the tap water in the cities can possibly be contaminated with germs.

If you don't have a taste for the water, you can also cover your fluid requirements with an unsweetened herbal tea. There are even special base herb teas.

4. Far too much raw food
Of course, it's healthy to eat raw vegetables. Sometimes the intestines cannot digest them that well and it is stressed. That is why you should listen carefully to your own body. If raw vegetables are eaten and the result is pain or gas, then these foods are probably the wrong choice. They should rather be steamed beforehand.

Likewise, people with food intolerances and allergy sufferers should be careful when choosing raw foods. Here, too, pain can arise.

5. Eating at the wrong times
Many people are used to eating when they are hungry - day or night. During an alkaline cure, however, attention should be paid to the different digestion times of cooked food and raw food. If you eat raw food after a cooked meal, gas can develop. This is particularly the case with fruit and is to blame for the internal rhythm of the liver. After 2 p.m., this is only hindered by raw food. Digesting is much worse.

6. Late meals
An alkaline diet and eating too late do not go together at all. Shift workers in particular need to be aware of this. Anything eaten after 6 p.m. ends up as weight on the hips. The liver's metabolism is particularly active at night.

7. Not chewing well
You learn it from childhood - every meal should always be chewed thoroughly. This also has several advantages. First of all, digestion begins in the mouth and can be processed better in the intestine. In addition, there will also be a lot less gas. If you chew longer, you are much more likely to be full. Why? Long chewing is simply more strenuous.

By the way - if you eat smaller portions, it is easier to chew much more slowly and thoroughly.

8. Stress
It's hard to believe, but not only the wrong foods can form acid, but also too much stress. That is why it is advisable to treat yourself to small moments

of calm again and again. This can be, for example, a walk in the fresh air or a relaxing bath.

All over Europe there are more and more base fasting hotels.

Closing word

The alkaline diet is an extremely complex topic.
This diet arose a long time ago from theories about the acid-base balance in the body. Then you get sick quickly if it's not in balance.
But that's not the only benefit of the alkaline diet - general well-being will improve quickly and you can even shed a few pounds.
The following foods, for example, are basic and therefore allowed:

- fruit
- vegetables
- water

But, on the other hand, this is not allowed:

- nicotine
- alcohol
- coffee
- meat
- sweets

It will not be particularly easy to regulate the renunciation at the beginning of a treatment. Fortunately, there are a few tricks that can make the days of alkaline fasting more bearable. You should always drink a lot and exercise every now and then doesn't hurt either. Otherwise the magic word is - motivation.

The alkaline diet also has a lot in common with the vegan diet and can also be combined well with other diets. An example would be detox, i.e. detoxifying the body.
If you want to take such a base cure, you should inform yourself thoroughly in advance and through suitable basic recipes. Not only are they delicious, they are but also really healthy. You can find a few here in the book - some relating to the versatile avocado, for example.

But enough said - now you have to try it out for yourself.
Basic nutrition. Purposeful and certainly not disappointing.

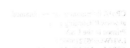